T0127739

Patient-Centered Care Series

Series Editors

Moira Stewart,
Judith Belle Brown
and
Thomas R Freeman

Chronic Myofascial Pain

A patient-centered approach

Edited by
Kirsti Malterud
and
Steinar Hunskaar

Radcliffe Medical Press

Radcliffe Medical Press Ltd
18 Marcham Road
Abingdon
Oxon OX14 1AA
United Kingdom

www.radcliffe-oxford.com
The Radcliffe Medical Press electronic catalogue and online ordering facility.
Direct sales to anywhere in the world.

———————————————————

© 2002 The authors

All rights reserved. No part of this publication may be reproduced, stored in
a retrieval system or transmitted, in any form or by any means, electronic,
mechanical, photocopying, recording or otherwise without the prior permis-
sion of the copyright owner.

British Library Cataloguing in Publication Data

A catalogue record for this book is available from the British Library.

ISBN 1 85775 947 8

Typeset by Aarontype Ltd, Easton, Bristol
Printed and bound by TJ International Ltd, Padstow, Cornwall

Contents

Series editors' introduction

The strength of medicine in curing many infectious diseases and some of the chronic diseases has also led to a key weakness. Some believe that medicine has abdicated its caring role and, in doing so, has not only alienated the public to some extent, but also failed to uphold its promise to 'do no harm'. One hears many stories of patients who have been technically cured but feel ill or who feel ill but for whom no satisfactory diagnosis is possible. In focusing so much attention on the nature of the disease, medicine has neglected the person who suffers the disease. Redressing this 20th century phenomenon required a new definition of medicine's role for the 21st century. A new clinical method, which has been developed during the 1980s and 1990s, has attempted to correct the flaw, to regain the balance between curing and caring. It is called a patient-centered clinical method and has been described and illustrated in *Patient-Centered Medicine: transforming the clinical method* (Stewart *et al.*, 1995) of which the 2nd edition is being prepared for publication in early 2003. In the 1995 book, conceptual, educational and research issues were elucidated in detail. The patient-centered conceptual framework from that book is used as the structure for each book in the series introduced here; it consists of six interactive components to be considered in every patient–practitioner interaction.

The first component is to assess the two modes of ill health; disease and illness. In addition to assessing the disease process, the clinician explores the patient's illness experience. Specifically, the practitioner considers how the patient feels about being ill, what the patient's ideas are about the illness, what impact the illness is having on the patient's functioning and what he or she expects from the clinician.

The second component is an integration of the concepts of disease and illness with an understanding of the whole person. This includes an awareness of the patient's position in the lifecycle and the social context in which they live.

The third component of the method is the mutual task of finding common ground between the patient and the practitioner. This consists of three key areas: mutually defining the problem, mutually defining the goals of management/treatment, and mutually exploring the roles to be assumed by the patient and the practitioner.

The fourth component is to use each visit as an opportunity for prevention and health promotion. The fifth component takes into consideration that each encounter with the patient should be used to develop the helping relationship;

the trust and respect that evolves in the relationship will have an impact on other components of the method. The sixth component requires that, throughout the process, the practitioner is realistic in terms of time, availability of resources and the amount of emotional and physical energy needed.

However, there is a gap between the description of the clinical method and its application in practice. The series of books presented here attempts to bridge that gap. Written by international leaders in their field, the series represents clinical explications of the patient-centered clinical method. Each volume deals with a common and challenging problem faced by practitioners. In each book, current thinking is organized in a similar way, reinforcing and illustrating the patient-centered clinical method. The common format begins with a description of the burden of illness, followed by chapters on the illness experience, the disease, the whole person, the patient–practitioner relationship and finding common ground, including current therapeutics.

The book series is international, to date representing Norway, Sweden, Canada, Australia, New Zealand and the USA. This is a testament to the universality of the values and concepts inherent in the patient-centered clinical method. The work of not only the authors, but others who have studied patients, has reinforced a virtually identical series of six components (Little *et al.*, 2001; Stewart, 2001). We feel that there is an emerging international definition of patient-centered practice which is represented in this book series.

The vigor of any clinical method is proven in the extent to which it is applicable in the clinical setting. It is anticipated that this series will inform further development of the clinical method and move thinking forward in this important aspect of medicine.

Moira Stewart PhD
Judith Belle Brown PhD
Thomas R Freeman MD, CCFP

References

Little P, Everitt H, Williamson I *et al.* (2001) Preferences of patients for patient-centred approach to consultation in primary care: observational study. *BMJ.* **322**(7284): 468–72.

Stewart M (2001) Towards a global definition of patient-centred care. *BMJ.* **322**(7284): 444–5.

Stewart M, Brown JB, Weston WW *et al.* (1995) *Patient-Centered Medicine: transforming the clinical method.* Sage Publications, Thousand Oaks, CA.

About the authors

Terje Alræk began his studies in acupuncture in 1978. Since graduating in Acupuncture at the International College of Oriental Medicine, England, in 1982, he has been in private practice. In 1997, he graduated in Chinese Herbal Medicine. Since 1994 he has been involved in research on complementary medicine, mainly on acupuncture effects on recurrent cystitis in adult women. He is now working 60% of his time as a research fellow at the University of Bergen, Norway.

Rae Frances Bell BA Hons, MD, a specialist in anesthesiology, is a senior consultant at the Department of Anesthesia and Intensive Care at Haukeland University Hospital in Bergen. Since 1994 she has been director of Norway's first multidisciplinary pain clinic which was established in 1985. She is leader of the Norwegian Society of Anesthesiologists' Advisory Committee on Pain. She is a member of the International Association for the Study of Pain (IASP), the Scandinavian Association for the Study of Pain (SASP) and the Pain Society of Great Britain and Ireland. Dr Bell is interested in many aspects of pain, including opioids and mechanisms of opioid tolerance and the treatment of neuropathic cancer pain. She is also interested in the integration of multidisciplinary knowledge and in the work of the multidisciplinary team with regard to all types of problematic pain.

Søren Brage MD, PhD, B Soc Sc is Associate Professor of Social Insurance Medicine, Department of General Practice and Community Medicine, University of Oslo, Norway. After 16 years of full-time general practice, he went into university studies, research and teaching. He holds part-time positions as Chief Medical Officer of the National Insurance Administration and as research fellow of the National Low Back Network, and is a member of the WONCA International Classification Committee. His dissertation was an epidemiological study on musculoskeletal disorders and their consequences for sickness absence. His present field of study is the epidemiology of chronic low back pain, including healthcare utilization and use of social security.

Dag Bruusgaard MD, PhD is Professor of Community Medicine and Chair at the Department of General Practice and Community Medicine, University of Oslo,

Norway. He is a part-time general practitioner, one of the founders of academic general practice in Norway, and former chairman of the European General Practice Research Workshop. He is involved in a variety of research projects in general practice and community medicine, focusing mainly on the epidemiology of musculoskeletal complaints and on social insurance medicine.

Lucy M Candib MD is a family physician who has taught and practiced family medicine, including obstetrics, in an urban neighborhood health center in Worcester, Massachusetts, USA, for the past 25 years. This health center is a residency training site within the Family Practice Residency Program of the University of Massachusetts where she is a Professor of Family Medicine and Community Health. Within the context of long-term doctor–patient relationships, Dr Candib has put feminist principles to work in a multicultural setting. She has also focused attention on the concerns of women trainees and practitioners in her work with family practice residents. She has lectured widely on the topics of sexual abuse and violence against women. She has introduced a feminist critique of medical theory in numerous articles and in her book, *Medicine and the Family: a feminist perspective* (1995). In 1995 she received a Fulbright grant to teach family medicine in Ecuador.

Hans-Jacob Haga MD, PhD is Professor and Consultant of Rheumatology, Centre for Rheumatic Diseases, University of Oslo, Norway. He has previously been Professor of Rheumatology at the Universities of Tromsø and Bergen, and President of the Norwegian and Scandinavian Societies for Rheumatology. His field of research is clinical and immunological studies of connective tissue diseases such as systemic lupus erythematosus, Sjögren's syndrome and vasculitis. His list of publications includes a variety of articles about clinical and immunological aspects of inflammatory rheumatic disorders, in addition to articles about patient satisfaction and quality aspects of diagnosis and treatment of rheumatic disorders. He has also written chapters in textbooks covering rheumatic disorders.

Katarina Hamberg MD, PhD is a specialist in family medicine. She is working part-time as a family physician at Mariehem's Health Center and part-time as Assistant Professor at the Faculty of Medicine, Umeå University, Umeå, Sweden. Since 1993 she has been working on the elaboration of a new development in medical education, professional development as a physician, which is focused on the consultation, theories and practical training of empathy and self-reflection. Her research deals with the problems facing patients and doctors when the patient suffers from biomedically unexplained symptoms, the patient–doctor relationship, gender bias in research and clinical work, and the role of biology and culture in the construction of gender identification in the individual. She has also published articles on scientific rigor in qualitative research.

Liv Haugli MD, PhD, MOH is a specialist in occupational medicine and is working as a research fellow at the Department of General Practice and Community Medicine, University of Oslo, Norway. Her field of research deals with developing and evaluating a group-learning program for persons with chronic musculoskeletal pain based on a phenomenological frame of understanding. She also works part-time as an occupational physician.

Steinar Hunskaar MD, PhD is Professor of Family Medicine, Department of Public Health and Primary Health Care, University of Bergen, Norway. He is also an approved specialist in family medicine and works part-time as a family physician. His main field of research deals with urinary incontinence in women, especially epidemiology, treatment and management in general practice. His thesis from 1987 dealt with spinal pain mechanisms and the mode of action of analgesic drugs. He has published numerous articles about pain, urinary incontinence and other clinical topics from a primary healthcare perspective. He has also edited a large Norwegian textbook of family medicine.

Eva E Johansson BA (Psychology), MD, PhD is working as a family physician in a healthcare center in Umeå, Sweden. Her interest in research evolved from experiences of difficult consultations, and she has taken an interest in issues such as illness perception, symptom presentation, and doctor–patient interaction in consultations. Findings from a qualitative research project are summarized in Dr Johansson's medical dissertation thesis, *Beyond Frustration: understanding women with undefined musculoskeletal pain who consult primary care*. Her research emphasizes the importance of a gender perspective in medicine. Since 1998 she has been engaged in research on gender bias in medicine – in medical education, clinical decision making and research. She is a part-time researcher and lecturer at the Department of Public Health and Clinical Medicine, Umeå University.

Alice Kvale PT, MSc is presently working as a research fellow and lecturer in the Section of Physiotherapy Research, University of Bergen, Norway. She has many years of clinical experience with multidisciplinary evaluation and treatment of patients with long-lasting pain problems. Her field of interest deals with the heterogeneous group of patients with long-lasting musculoskeletal pain problems. Her present research focuses on physiotherapy examinations related to posture, movement, muscle, skin and respiration.

Kirsti Malterud MD, PhD is Professor of Family Medicine, Department of Public Health and Primary Health Care, University of Bergen, Norway. She works part-time as a family physician, and also holds a part-time position as Professor of Family Medicine, University of Copenhagen, Denmark. Her field of research deals with women's health, medical communication and the theory of medicine and science. Her extensive list of publications includes a variety of articles about medically unexplained disorders in women, and the insufficiency of medical theory and practice to include the knowledge held by the patients themselves about their health problems. She has also written an introductory book and several articles about the use of qualitative methods in medical research.

Halvard Nilsen MD is a consultant in rehabilitation medicine at the Department of Physical Medicine and Rehabilitation, Ålesund Central Hospital, Norway. He is also a specialist in clinical social medicine and educated in psychosomatic medicine. He works with rehabilitation of people with pain syndromes in multidisciplinary teams. He has much experience from postgraduate teaching and projects in rehabilitation and pain treatment. He is now mainly focused on the clinical work; how to combine somatic knowledge with understanding of the patients' experiences in order to make good individual treatment plans. Dr Nilsen has a broad clinical background from related fields such as geriatric medicine, psychiatry, insurance medicine, occupational medicine, trauma rehabilitation and cardiology.

Eldri Steen RN, PhD is a research fellow and an adviser for the Norwegian Resource Center for Rheumatological Rehabilitation at The Deaconess Hospital, Oslo. Her field of research deals with developing and evaluating a group-learning program for persons with chronic musculoskeletal pain based on a phenomenological frame of understanding.

Per Stensland MD gained his experience as a family physician in rural districts in northern and western Norway, and has been working as a Senior District Medical Officer in Botswana for two years. He has been a member of the board of the Norwegian College of General Practitioners for six years and is the leader of the International Committee of the College. He holds a part-time position as Associate Professor of Family Medicine, Department of Public Health and Primary Health Care, University of Bergen, Norway. His field of research deals with the challenge of understanding and finding treatment for patients suffering from long-standing illness without clinical findings.

Arne Tjølsen MD, PhD is Professor of Physiology, University of Bergen, Norway. He is now at the Department of Neurology, Bergen University Hospital, and part-time at the Department of Physiology, University of Bergen. His main research interest is the changing sensitivity in pain pathways in the central nervous system. The research includes studies of the descending modulatory systems to the spinal cord, and mechanisms for long-term increase of pain sensitivity. Such mechanisms are probably active in long-lasting or chronic pain conditions. The most recent focus has been on mechanisms for long-term changes that are similar to the basic mechanisms thought to be important in

learning and memory. His research has been presented in a series of international publications, and he has written several book chapters on the neurophysiology of pain.

Nina K Vøllestad PhD is Professor of Health Science, Faculty of Medicine, University of Oslo, Norway. Her basic training is in physiology, with special interest
and research background in muscle physiology and motor control. Her field of
interest over the last 10 years has been work-related musculoskeletal injury
and pain. Over the last couple of years, her research has also included rehabilitation. She has an extensive list of publications, including papers dealing with
mechanisms of muscle fatigue and how muscle activation is related to muscle
pain. She is also involved in research on classification of functioning of patients
in various settings.

Introduction

Patients with medically unexplained disorders are well known to the family physician. These patients suffer from long-standing and often disabling subjective symptoms, although objective findings are lacking. Causal explanations may seem complex or cloudy, and contemporary biomedical frameworks offer no simple or universal solutions for understanding and management.

Relating to patients with medically unexplained disorders, typically exemplified by those who suffer from chronic myofascial pain, represents a great challenge to the healthcare provider. What are we supposed to do when we, as the patients' healthcare providers, realize that we are not able to relieve their pain, perhaps not even able to share their understanding of the problems? These are not the kind of problems that medical school taught us to solve. Unchecked, the difficulty of the situation may be transformed to the patient, who runs a risk of being labelled as a difficult patient. Not only is her body in pain, her burden of suffering may be increased when those who were supposed to help her seem to distrust her or work against her.

It is our belief as editors of this book that family medicine has seriously failed in its medical responsibility if it cannot accommodate this group of patients in a professional way. This is partly a matter of knowledge, partly a matter of attitudes, but perhaps most of all a matter of values and relationships. These elements, constituting the foundations of clinical practice, deserve to be expounded and elaborated for the purpose of good quality practice.

The patient-centered clinical method (PCCM) has, in the last few decades, earned an incontestable position as the foundation for clinical practice and research in family medicine in Scandinavia and worldwide. Patients' perspectives are now increasingly implemented in clinical medicine in general. Inspired by the significant work initiated by Professor Ian R McWhinney and co-workers at the Center for Studies in Family Medicine, The University of Western Ontario, we have had the great pleasure to become acquainted with the theoretical framework of the patient-centered clinical method. The principles and procedures of this approach seem to be tailored to the demanding and rewarding context of patient–provider encounters in primary care, perhaps especially suited for the care of patients with long-standing, chronic illness. At the Section for General Practice, University of Bergen, Norway, patient-centered medicine has been a key-stone in teaching and research for many years. We have developed undergraduate courses showing medical students how to practice the method during clinical work, and we have promoted the method in postgraduate courses and CME activities. Clinical research and theoretical projects have been shaped by the thinking and practice of patient-centered medicine.

We want to express our gratitude to the London, Ontario, group for this inspiration, as well as for their invitation to join this book series on the clinical application of the patient-centered approach. A brief look into our own experiences from practice and research made us conclude that we would use this opportunity to assemble knowledge that could be used in encounters with patients suffering from chronic myofascial pain. To us, this group of patients constituted the most obvious context for elaborating and discussing the features, strengths and pitfalls of the patient-centered clinical method. We appreciated this opportunity to shift attention from models, guidelines and teaching checklists to challenges occurring when the method is utilized in real-life situations where time schedules may be brief, patients may be desperate and physicians may feel helpless.

This book is not written as a comprehensive textbook intended to cover all you need to know about chronic myofascial pain. Within the overall frame of the book series, we have chosen to present certain selected topics, assuming these to provide inspiration and enthusiasm for further reading and development. Our approach emphasizes investigation, management and support when no clear-cut biomedical explanation of the pain is found. We pursue the emotional and professional challenges these conditions place upon the physician. Conditions related to acute pain, pain related to specific medical diseases, cancer pain and pain in palliative care are not dealt with in this volume. We have focused on pain in adult patients, and excluded pain syndromes in children and adolescents.

To facilitate the application of the knowledge presented in the book, and to emphasize the patient perspective, we invented Mrs Judith Smith, whom you will first meet in Chapter 1, and then follow all through the book. She represents a summarized experience of patients we have met, and has been given the task of providing a personal face and image of patients suffering from chronic myofascial pain. We thank all the Mrs Smiths we met during the years in our practices for sharing with us their experiences of suffering and strength.

Editing this volume of the book series has been a pleasure, thanks to the fertile soil of research and experience found in our closest neighborhood. We have been able to draw on an ample network of potential authors in Norway and abroad, who enthusiastically and unanimously accepted our requests to present and share their knowledge with colleagues in this book. One of the authors, Lucy Candib, generously offered important contributions beyond her authorship by polishing the language of several chapters.

In Chapter 1, Bruusgaard and Brage recapitulate the concept and proportion of chronic myofascial pain as part of the broad field of musculoskeletal disorders. Empirical research is presented, describing the magnitude of the problem, the part of illness that leads to medical care, the distribution of various pain syndromes in family medicine, regional differences in prevalences and welfare consequences. Chapter 2 deals with basic pain mechanisms on neurophysiology and muscle physiology (Tjølsen and Vøllestad), prevailing multidimensional models for clinical understanding of chronic pain syndromes (Bell) and clinical and laboratory examination for patients with chronic pain (Haga).

The first component of the patient-centered clinical model requires the physician to explore both the disease and the illness experience. In Chapter 3, Stensland approaches the meaning and impact of the illness experience by sharing narratives and experiences from a qualitative study where he used home notes like a diary to facilitate the communication of illness experience. Johansson and Hamberg supplement the picture by presenting findings from an interview study with women sick-listed for medically unexplained pain conditions. These authors offer a gender lens as a tool for broader understanding of the illness experience in a group of patients where women constitute the majority. The second component of the patient-centered clinical model is an integrated understanding of the whole person, including the patient's individual development, family lifecycle and social context. These matters are pursued by Johansson and Hamberg in Chapter 4, where they present challenges related to family, work, health and rehabilitation for women patients, elucidated by their study. This chapter also includes Candib's review of the multiple layers of oppression in culture, family and healthcare that may cause, worsen or surround the pain problems. The fifth component of the patient-centered clinical model, conscious attention to enhancing the patient–clinician relationship, is dealt with in Chapter 5, where Hamberg and Johansson again draw from their interview study to illustrate the relational challenges emerging when things go wrong and the patient feels turned down and distrusted. Malterud presents empowering approaches from her research within this field, where the discourse is reframed by key questions inviting the patient to reveal her agenda and attend to her strengths. In Chapter 6, experts from different fields demonstrate various tools for management and coping, suggesting that diversity may be a prerequisite for the third and the sixth component of the patient-centered clinical method – finding common ground and being realistic. Nilsen writes about medical treatment, Stensland returns with suggestions about an illness diary as a method for changing the discourse, and Kvale presents perspectives on cross-disciplinary approaches and physiotherapy, supplemented by Candib on massage therapies. Haugli and Steen share their experiences from a group-learning program, as an example of occupational rehabilitation approaches, and Alraek discusses the contributions of complementary medicine by discussing Chinese medicine and acupuncture. Malterud closes the chapter by sharing a model for recovery, where positive views of the future are sustained by attention to acknowledgment and hope.

Medical practice within the area of non-malignant chronic pain has so far largely been based upon unsystematized experiential knowledge. In this volume,

we have combined common sense, patient-centered and evidence-based perspectives, as they can be applied in the busy, everyday life of clinical practice.
The point of departure of the book is to regard chronic pain as an essentially
subjective and experienced phenomenon, taking place in the life and body of
a particular human being, living in a specific sociocultural context. The family physician's task is to gain an understanding of the symptom, its origins,
consequences, and meanings for the person in question. By combining this par-
ticularized knowledge with the best available evidence about diagnosis and
treatment of this kind of pain, it may be possible to overcome the shortcomings
of contemporary biomedicine in explaining and resolving these kinds of illnesses. After all, the essential principles of PCCM, which constitute assigning
privilege to the patient's perspective, researching parallel agendas, and finding
common ground, represent a value commitment. We believe this commitment
cannot be adequately accounted for unless the physician takes responsibility
and challenges the inequality of power that is inherent in the patient–provider
relationship.

The authors finished their manuscripts in Spring 2000. Due to different circumstances beyond our control, the process of producing this book has taken
some time. We are now happy to share the text with readers.

Kirsti Malterud
Steinar Hunskaar
Bergen, Norway
June 2002

The magnitude of the problem

Dag Bruusgaard and Søren Brage

Mrs Judith Smith, aged 55, has for the last 15 years been suffering from steadily increasing pain in her chest and shoulders. In recent years, her feet have also been terrible after a long day at work. She has taken painkillers for periods of time, but never finds any long-term relief from medication. The last few months, Judith Smith has felt exhausted with no energy whatsoever, but still kept on doing her work at the hospital laundry, where she has worked for the last 19 years. She has problems falling asleep, and during the night she is not able to get a good rest. She dreams a lot and wakes up with her head filled with worries and pain. Although her heart sometimes gives her palpitations, she does not really believe that the chest pain comes from her heart. However, her mother died from a heart attack, so she is somewhat concerned. She feels that strain at work and at home increases her muscular tension, but she is not able to change her situation and relieve her symptoms.

Yesterday, Judith Smith received a 20-page questionnaire from a research group, who knew that she had been sick-listed within the last year due to pain problems. She is puzzled about what to answer, when the researchers instruct her to choose between boxes of respectively widespread or localized pain. Actually, the pain is just all over, although it may differ from day to day. She also wonders whether she should agree to the suggestion that this is a chronic condition, because she desperately hopes that sooner or later she will get rid of her problems.

The problem

Symptoms from the musculoskeletal system are reasons for reduced quality of life for a substantial part of the population. They represent a great burden to society because of reduced working capacity, sick leave and disability pensions, and they are problematic for the healthcare system as a result of insufficient means to prevent and treat the conditions.

The concept of chronic myofascial pain

There is a confusing magnitude of names given to musculoskeletal pain complaints, reflecting diverging opinions and a lack of consensus on what it is all about. The International Classification of Diseases, latest edition (ICD 10), illustrates the problem of classifying unspecific and widespread musculoskeletal complaints (Box 1.1). They are situated in two different chapters.

Under Chapter M, 'Diseases of the musculoskeletal system and connective tissue', we have to go down to M79, 'Other soft-tissue disorders, not elsewhere classified, excluding: soft-tissue pain, psychogenic (F 45.4)'. Here we will find M79.0, 'Rheumatism, unspecified', which includes fibromyalgia and fibrositis. Chronic widespread muscle-pain syndromes should be included under this chapter, although not stated explicitly. Otherwise, if the musculoskeletal origin is questioned, generalized pain might be registered under Chapter R, 'Symptoms, signs and abnormal clinical or laboratory findings, not elsewhere classified'. Under R52, 'Pain, not elsewhere classified' we find R52.9, 'Pain unspecified, including generalized pain, not otherwise specified' at the very end of the pain section.

The ICD chapter on diseases of the musculoskeletal system and connective tissue does not include injuries, tumors and malformations; however, these

---

Box 1.1 *International classification of diseases ICD 10*

- *Chapter M: Diseases of the musculoskeletal system and connective tissue*

  - M79 Other soft tissue disorders, not elsewhere classified, excluding soft tissue pain, psychogenic (F 45.4)
  - M79.0 Rheumatism, unspecified

- *Chapter R: Symptoms, signs and abnormal clinical or laboratory findings, not elsewhere classified*

  - R52 Pain, not elsewhere classified
  - R52.9 Pain unspecified, including generalized pain, not otherwise specified

conditions are included in the chapter on musculoskeletal health problems in the International Classification for Primary Health Care (ICPC).

The International Association for the Study of Pain (IASP) suggests in the second edition from 1994 (Merskey and Bogduk, 1994) a detailed classification of chronic pain with five axes based on region, system, temporal characteristics, intensity and etiology. According to their definitions, fibromyalgia is classified as a 'relatively generalized syndrome' in the musculoskeletal system. They make a note to distinguish fibromyalgia from chronic myofascial pain (CMP) because they consider that the concept of myofascial pain syndromes also might include localized muscular pain. They also include what they call 'Pain of psychological origin', subdivided into:

- muscle tension
- delusional or hallucinatory
- hysterical, conversion, or hypochondriacal
- associated with depression.

IASP, in its focusing on pain, does not include chronic widespread pain (CWP) as a condition reaching further than fibromyalgia. Overall, the contribution from ICD and IASP to the classification and understanding of the CMP syndromes is limited. For the purpose of this chapter, a possible simple classification, focusing on the musculoskeletal system, could be:

- strain-related musculoskeletal complaints, including soft-tissue rheumatism, both localized as tendinitis and myalgia, and widespread as CMP and fibromyalgia
- inflammatory musculoskeletal complaints, including rheumatoid arthritis and ankylosing spondylitis (AS)
- degenerative musculoskeletal complaints, including osteoporosis and osteoarthritis
- other musculoskeletal complaints, including injuries, deformities, infections and tumors.

One problem with this grouping is where to put the chronic low back pain conditions. They are often considered strain related, but, on x-ray, have at the same time frequently degenerative signs. Textbooks include mostly the latter three categories, while the first one affects the greatest number of persons. In this chapter, we will focus on this first category, on what we have called the strain-related conditions, in particular CWP.

Chronic widespread pain includes fibromyalgia, but reaches further than the fibromyalgia concept. We will use the American College of Rheumatology's (ACR) definition of fibromyalgia (Wolfe *et al.*, 1990), if not stated explicitly otherwise. This definition is based on three dimensions:

- duration (at least three months)
- localization (widespread; that is, axial pain, pain on the left and right side, and pain above and below the waist)
- tender points (pain at 11 or more out of 18 specified anatomical locations).

Although the ACR definition is widely accepted and used, there is still a great controversy about the fibromyalgia concept. Some still claim that it is a distinct clinical entity with specific causes needing specific treatment, whilst others, including IASP, consider fibromyalgia at one extreme of a continuous spectrum of distress and pain, starting with localized complaints of short duration, and ending with chronic widespread complaints.

There is no commonly accepted definition of CMP. One solution to the lack of definition is to use the ACR definition without the tender-point criterion. A group in Manchester, UK, has suggested an alternative definition of widespread pain, hereafter referred to as CWP(M). For subjects to satisfy the definition, pain must be reported in at least two sections in each of two contralateral limbs and in the axial skeleton. CMP is first and foremost an epidemiological term, reflecting self-reported, long-lasting, widespread complaints of suspected muscular origin, while fibromyalgia is a term based on a clinical examination. In this chapter, we will use CMP synonymously with CWP.

The prevalence of musculoskeletal complaints

Musculoskeletal complaints are frequent in the population. Earlier studies focused primarily on localized pain as low back pain or shoulder/neck pain, often in association with working conditions. When Yunus introduced criteria for the diagnosis of fibromyalgia (Yunus *et al.*, 1989), it opened a new area with focus also on widespread pain, a tendency supported by the ACR criteria. Such conditions are often called 'diffuse', in English often related to something that is spread, scattered and widespread as opposed to localized. In Norwegian 'diffuse' usually gives associations to something foggy or contourless, not to be grasped, clearly seen or even taken seriously.

Adults

A sample of the adult population in a Norwegian municipality received a mailed questionnaire, including the extensively used Nordic form on musculoskeletal complaints. 85.1% of 2361 responders reported pain or discomfort from at least one region of the body during the last 12 months (Natvig *et al.* 1994). Of the 10 regions marked on a body mannequin, low back (total 52.9%, female 54.7%, male 50.7%), head (total 48.9%, female 60.5%, male 36.3%), neck (total 47.9%, female 57.6%, male 37.3%), and shoulder (total 46.8%, female 56.2%, male 36.5%) were most frequently checked off.

15.3% of the 2361 responders reported daily symptoms during the whole year. Daily symptoms increased with age, and were more common among women than men. In women, the fraction reporting daily symptoms increased from 7.7% in the 20–22 year-old group, to a maximum of 30.9% in the 60–62 year-old group; the corresponding figures for men were 4.9% and 20.8%.

Persons reporting low back pain as part of widespread pain were more often women, had more chronic complaints, reported in general more discomfort and more functional limitations compared to the ones reporting low back pain as their only musculoskeletal complaint.

A population study in the UK found a crude prevalence of CWP to be 15.6% among women and 9.4% among men, using the ACR criteria for social prevelance of symptoms (Croft *et al.*, 1993). In contrast to most other studies, a study using the Manchester criteria did not find a statistically significant gender difference (5.3% among women and 3.7% among men) (Macfarlane *et al.*, 1996).

In a study of the population aged 40–42 in a Norwegian county, 7127 persons responded (62% response rate). During the preceding year, 73.8% of the women and 62.4% of the men reported musculoskeletal complaints, with an increasing gender gap the more chronic and widespread the complaints. 32.6% and 23.6% reported chronic pain (lasting for at least three months), 13.5% and 4.7% reported CWP (affecting at least five out of nine regions, bilateral counting as one), 3.0% and 0.1% respectively claimed to have the diagnosis of fibromyalgia, giving sex ratio of 1.18, 1.38, 2.87 and 30.0 respectively (Aarflot and Bruusgaard, 1994).

Some studies have found female prevalence of CWP as high as 20% (Macfarlane, 1999). The prevalence of CWP has thus varied substantially according to what definition has been used. In contrast to CWP where criteria are lacking, the ACR criteria for fibromyalgia have been internationally accepted. The ACR criteria have been used in several surveys that have included clinical examinations. Prevalence rates from 2% to 13% among women have been reported. The great variation in prevalence of fibromyalgia reflects methodological difficulties rather than real differences in prevalence of the conditions. Different interpretations of the tender-point criterion could partly explain the variation.

One general conclusion from all these studies is that the majority of subjects with chronic widespread musculoskeletal pain do not meet the present fibromyalgia criteria.

Children

All schoolchildren in a local community aged 10, 13 and 15 were given questionnaires to be filled in during an ordinary school session (Smedbråten *et al.*, 1998).

569 children answered (86.5% of all the pupils in the three age groups). They were asked if they *usually* felt pain anywhere in the body, regardless of location. Further, they were asked to register the pain on a map of the body. Here, 12 regions were marked and named, making no attempt to distinguish pain from the locomotor system from other types of pain.

73% answered 'yes' to the question of usually feeling pain, 82% of the girls and 64% of the boys. Knee, head and back were the regions most frequently reported. The number of regions reported was highest among girls, where it also increased with age. Among the ones reporting pain, 27% of the girls and 24% of the boys said they sometimes used medication for the symptoms.

Several studies among children, most of them from Scandinavia, showed the same high prevalence of the reporting of bodily pain (Kristjansdottir 1997; Mikkelsson *et al.*, 1997). One study from Israel found a high number of children meeting the ACR criteria for fibromyalgia, although the symptoms and signs varied more over time than what was usually seen in adult fibromyalgia patients (Buskila *et al.*, 1995).

Associated symptoms

Musculoskeletal pain has long been associated with other signs and symptoms, and Yunus required the existence of so-called minor criteria for the diagnosis of fibromyalgia (Yunus *et al.*, 1989). These features were fatigue, poor sleep, anxiety/depression, irritable bowel syndrome, headache, swelling in fingers or feet and numbness in fingers or feet. No accepted definition of these symptoms has been made, and the ACR did not keep the minor criteria in their definition of fibromyalgia. They did not find that these symptoms were helpful to distinguish fibromyalgia from other chronic pain conditions. Still, the association between fibromyalgia, CWP and the mentioned symptoms seems a reality, as the following data indicates.

In the previously cited study, the association between answers to questions about muscular complaints and simple *yes/no* questions on the existence of associated symptoms has been analyzed. These symptoms were prevalent among the 40–42 year-old respondents; any one of the seven symptoms was reported by 65.7% of the women and 47.7% of the men. Non-refreshed sleep was most frequently reported (women 34.7%, men 26.8%) (Aarflot, 1999).

There was a strong correlation between the number of painful sites and the number of reported symptoms, both in men and women. The mean number of painful sites increased linearly, from one out of nine among the ones not reporting any associated symptoms to almost seven among those reporting all seven symptoms (Figure 1.1). The proportion of women reporting a diagnosis of fibromyalgia rose exponentially from almost nil among those without associated

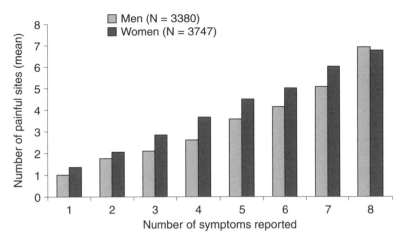

Figure 1.1 Number of symptoms and painful sites. Men and women. Oestfold County, Norway (Aarflot 1999).

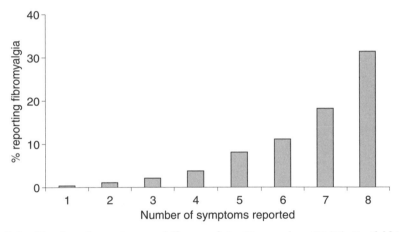

Figure 1.2 Number of symptoms and fibromyalgia. Women ($n = 3747$). Oestfold County, Norway (Aarflot 1999).

symptoms to 31.6% among those reporting all seven symptoms (Figure 1.2). When comparing women with fibromyalgia with those with CWP, fibromyalgia excluded, only fatigue was more frequent in women with self-reported fibromyalgia when controlling for the number of painful sites. This study also found an increasing prevalence of CWP (gout excluded) with increasing levels of uric acid, and that women with CWP more often had thyroid microsomal antibodies than controls without such complaints. These findings, also found in a Swedish study, have still to be confirmed, but could be explained as part of a multisymptom syndrome.

The association between mental distress, sleep problems, and bodily pain has also been found among children. The association to most pain localizations, except knees, was found, and there was also an increased association with a greater number of regions affected (Bruusgaard *et al.*, 2000).

Sex and age

We have documented that bodily pain is frequent in the population, children and adults alike. Empirical studies show that the more chronic and widespread, the greater the female dominance. The finding of a moderate, statistically insignificant gender difference in CWP in the Manchester study has to be supported from other studies to really question this statement.

The great leap in the gender ratio between CWP and fibromyalgia *might* be an indication that they are really different conditions, but could as well be the result of the diagnostic process. Fibromyalgia-like conditions are not expected among men, and might not be reported by men even when they exist. Practitioners' reporting of fibromyalgia-like conditions being frequent among immigrant men is an interesting observation. So far, this clinical observation has not been sustained from systematic inquiries.

Chronic pain seems to increase with age, while CWP seems to be most frequent among persons in the age group 40–60. This might reflect a true decrease in CWP in the elderly, but might also be a cohort phenomenon, with age-dependent differences in reporting behavior.

Natural history and variations in time and place

There is no good support for the claim that CWP conditions are increasing in industrialized societies. Data from the Norwegian national health surveys may indicate a slightly increasing tendency. The magnitude of the increase, however, is so small that it might just reflect minor changes in reporting behavior.

Few long-term follow-up studies have been performed. Still, we do not know how many of the children reporting long-lasting complaints will end up as permanent, adult sufferers. A lack of association between childhood and adult complaints seems an unreasonable assumption. Although fibromyalgia-like conditions among children seem to vary to a great extent, the findings in adults so far indicate that the more widespread the complaints, and the more associated the symptoms, the more stable and unchanging the situation. Established fibromyalgia seems to be a permanent condition, although fluctuating from time to time. Board members of the Norwegian Fibromyalgia Association (NFA) have claimed that in a situation where fibromyalgia goes into total remission, one should question the diagnosis.

It is believed that musculoskeletal complaints are more prevalent in northern Europe, with its harsh climate and strict and regulated societies, compared to Mediterranean countries which have warmer climates and more relaxed life-styles. At least, these conditions are less frequently reported in Mediterranean countries than in the Nordic countries. In the US, such complaints seem more frequent among Caucasians than Blacks and people of Hispanic origin (Smythe, 1985). Likewise, musculoskeletal complaints have been seen as the result of a modern, sedentary lifestyle. Contrary to this is the fact that in Botswana, a condition called 'total body pain' is a frequent cause for consulting primary healthcare, and in rural South Africa, fibromyalgia seems to occur as frequently as in industrialized countries.

Etiology

There has been much controversy over the etiology of musculoskeletal com-plaints in general, and CWP in particular. Fibromyalgia and other unspecific conditions have, by some, been seen as a hysterical construct, as artificial non-sense. An editorial in the *Journal of Psychosomatic Medicine* in 1995 ironically introduced the term 'the disease of the month' relating to conditions like fibro-myalgia and chronic fatigue syndrome (CFS) (Shorter, 1995).

Much focus has been placed on the association between mental distress, sleep problems and fibromyalgia. The discussion has been on whether this associa-tion is a causal one, and in which direction. There is no doubt that chronic pain causes mental distress and sleep difficulties. Some evidence exists that it is also the other way round, that sleep problems might provoke muscular ten-sion and pain, and that muscular pain might be a result of mental distress in general and depression in particular. Recent studies indicate that both sleep problems and CMP are indicators of general discomfort and predictors of future functional limitations. Until the last few decades, focus has been on the relation-ship between such complaints and working conditions, and expressions such as 'work-related musculoskeletal complaints' have been used. For a period, there was a strong belief in ergonomic work site approaches to prevent and treat musculoskeletal complaints. The results have, however, been marginal and hence disappointing.

It seems reasonable, though, that complaints from the locomotor system could be the result of physical or mental strain, from overuse, underuse or incorrect use of the locomotor system. Results so far substantiate the causal relation-ship between strain and musculoskeletal complaints (Bernhard, 1997). Should anyone be in doubt, just look at athletes and ballet dancers. They are at the top extreme of physical strain in the workplace, resulting in almost inevitable musculoskeletal complaints.

From population studies, the striking find is, however, how little occupational strain is able to explain the variation in prevalence. Of localized pain, both neck/shoulder pain and low back pain are associated with occupational factors, while widespread pain can hardly be explained by conditions in the workplace.

A consistent finding is that the prevalence of widespread pain increases with decreasing length of education and decreasing social status. The few studies on genetic factors show, not surprisingly, that the heterogeneous group of unexplained musculoskeletal conditions are partly genetically determined.

Firm conclusions as to the etiology of conditions prevalent in the population might come up against problems where exact knowledge is missing. The rise and fall of the repetitive strain injury (RSI) epidemic in Australia clearly demonstrates this (Barton, 1989). Upper limb/shoulder/neck complaints were considered as occupational injuries. The healthcare system and the labor organizations focused strongly on the condition, and the sufferers were entitled to insurance benefits. This resulted in a dramatic rise in the recording of these conditions. A court decision questioned the association, with the following withdrawal of benefits and decline in the epidemic. This incident has given support to the theory that musculoskeletal pain complaints, and other medically unexplained conditions, might partly be a cultural phenomenon. This opens the possibility that CWP might be the result of learned behavior, with the possibility of spreading like contagious disease epidemics.

Of the many other associations, and hence possible causal factors, to have been found, one requires mention here. Smokers have more pain in general, and low back pain in particular, than non-smokers, even when controlling for some possible confounders, such as physical and mental strain.

Chronic myofascial pain: part of a multisymptom syndrome?

Some authors have been fascinated by the similarity between a number of the most controversial pain and discomfort conditions, including fibromyalgia and chronic fatigue syndrome. Ursin (1997) put these conditions into four symptom categories:

- muscle pain
- gastrointestinal problems

- allergies/colds
- pseudoneurological complaints (fatigue, dizziness, vertigo, anxiety, depressed mood and sleep disturbance).

He suggests lumping the conditions together rather than looking at them as separate entities. Clauw and Chrousos (1997) have established the hypothesis that genetic and environmental factors interact in developing such multisymptom syndromes through a common pathway, a central nervous system dysfunction. Theoretically, the cause might be biological stressors as well as psychosocial ones affecting particularly vulnerable persons, or the sum of several stressors ending up in a situation intolerable for the affected individual, whether they have an increased vulnerability or not. This might help to explain the finding of an association between chronic pain, a series of signs and symptoms of discomfort and some biological parameters. If such hypotheses gain support from future research, one implication would be to focus less on the musculoskeletal system, and rather look upon CWP as one of several indications of disturbed bodily functions. For the patients, the CMP is often the most bothering symptom, and hence the symptom most frequently presented to the doctor. Some patients with chronic widespread musculoskeletal pain, including fibromyalgia, might thus have a multisymptom syndrome. Perhaps we should reintroduce other signs and symptoms of discomfort in the definition. It might be that such symptoms are more important than the tender-point criterion.

The problem of the lack of criterion for CMP, and criteria for fibromyalgia with varying interpretation, will not be solved with reintroduction of associated symptoms. The multisymptom syndrome approach might, however, be a fruitful way forward in the understanding of CMP. If so, we need to differentiate between the patients with multiple localized complaints and those with transient problems. A duration of three months, as in the ACR criteria, seems, in any case, to be too short. A solution could be to avoid redefinition of the criteria until our knowledge and understanding of the complaints is better. In retrospect, one could question the enthusiasm with which the ACR criteria were met. The strong focus on tender points might have been misleading in the process of better understanding these conditions.

The consequences of chronic myofascial pain

For the individual, the most important consequences of CMP are limitations of daily life functions and reduced work ability. For society as a whole, the utilization of health services and generated healthcare costs are the most-studied consequences of the disease. CMP is a strain on the public economy, and causes great controversy with respect to the awarding of disability benefits.

Most research on the epidemiology of CMP has been completed on clinical populations. Thus, the prevalence of its consequences in the general population can only be estimated indirectly from what is known about the consequences of musculoskeletal disorders (MSDs) in general, and of fibromyalgia in particular. As mentioned previously, MSDs refer to disorders in muscle, bone, joints and connective tissue. The ICD has most frequently been used to classify this group of disorders, and comparisons between studies are therefore possible. It should be noted, however, that injuries to the musculoskeletal system are sometimes included, sometimes not.

Functional limitation

In Canada, USA and Western Europe, MSDs cause more functional limitations in the adult population than any other group of disorders. In the Ontario Health Survey (Badley et al., 1994), they caused 40% of all chronic conditions, 54% of all long-term disability, and 24% of all restricted activity days. The prevalence of disabilities due to MSDs has repeatedly been estimated to be 4%–5% of adult populations (Reynolds et al., 1992). It is higher in women, and increases strongly with age.

The disabling consequences of the MSDs were estimated in detail in a Canadian study. The prevalence of disability due to arthritis/rheumatism was 2.7%, disability due to back disorders was 1.6%, trauma 0.4%, bone disorders 0.1%, and disability due to 'other' MSDs was 0.5% (Reynolds et al., 1992). It is probable that the group 'other' included CMP syndromes. It seems reasonable, on the basis of these and other studies, to assume that the most common causes of musculoskeletal-related disability are osteoarthritis, rheumatoid arthritis and low back disorders. However, CMP also causes disability in a considerable number of individuals, but the precise magnitude remains to be settled.

Disability is more severe in fibromyalgia patients than in patients with other musculoskeletal conditions or in controls (White et al., 1999). Nevertheless, the severity of disability shows large variations. Studies on fibromyalgia patients have demonstrated considerable limitations of function and work ability in the more severely ill, but also that the majority of these patients have fair functional level, and manage to stay at work. A study including 81 fibromyalgia patients showed that they worked more hours than the American average, and more than half of the patients did not report any work days lost in the previous year (Cathey et al., 1986). A relatively small group of patients had considerable absence, and accounted for the majority of days lost.

Work disability

Work disability is a much-studied consequence of MSDs. The ability to work is linked to self-realization, more secure social position and improved quality of life. A chronic pain condition might lead to temporary, recurrent or permanent loss of work ability. Temporary and recurrent disability in the economically active population might be the consequence in milder cases, and can be explored in registers on sickness absence (sick leave) or workers' compensation claims. Permanent disability, on the other hand, can be estimated on the basis of disability pensions' registers.

When examining studies on the consequences of MSDs on work disability, one is struck by the variation in published results. The explanations for this variation are several. First of all, disability benefit schemes have different levels of compensation and rates are, quite naturally, higher in welfare states that give more generous benefits. National or local criteria for pensions and sick leave, e.g. minimum length of employment, also vary greatly and affect the rates.

A second main obstacle lies in the conceptualization in different studies and countries. As mentioned earlier, overall rates for MSDs can often be compared. However, subgroups are not uniformly defined in the literature. This holds true in particular for conditions where the diagnosis, such as CMP and fibromyalgia, mainly has to be based on the patients' symptoms, and where there is no agreement on etiology. In many countries, e.g. in Norway, CMP is rarely used as a diagnosis. Instead, fibromyalgia, soft-tissue disorder, general muscle pain or pain syndrome is used.

Sick leave

MSDs cause a major part of all sickness absence, as experienced in Scandinavia (Tellnes *et al.*, 1989), Poland (Szubert *et al.*, 1997), UK, and USA. In short-term sickness absence (less than one to two weeks), they are second only to respiratory disorders. For long-term absence, which is more important than short-term absence for the individual in terms of consequences, and for society in terms of costs, musculoskeletal injuries and disorders are the most common medical causes. They cause more than half of all sickness absence longer than two weeks in Norway (Brage *et al.*, 1998).

It is not possible to determine precisely how large a fraction of the musculoskeletal-related sickness absence is caused by CMP, but probably the fraction is small. Sickness absence statistics from Norway show that 1.5% of persons on sick leave due to MSDs have been given the diagnoses muscle pain or fibromyalgia (Brage *et al.*, 1998) (Table 1.1). It is probable that some patients with CMP are given other diagnoses than fibromyalgia.

Table 1.1 Distribution (in percent) of persons with sick leave longer than 14 days due to musculoskeletal and connective tissue disorders by diagnosis and gender, Norway, 1994 (based on Brage *et al.*, 1998).

Diagnosis	Men N= 75 228	Women N= 81 416	Total N= 156 644
Low back disorders	35	31	33
Neck and shoulder disorders	16	23	20
Musculoskeletal injuries	23	12	17
Tendinitis, epicondylitis, ganglion	6	7	7
Rheumatoid arthritis	3	3	3
Osteoarthritis	2	2	2
Muscle pain/fibromyalgia	0.5	2.4	1.5
Other musculoskeletal disorders (MSDs)	15	19	17
Sum	**100**	**100**	**100**

Disability pension

As for temporary benefits, MSDs are also common causes for disability pensions. Other frequent causes are mental disorders, including mental retardation, and cardiovascular disorders. The relative importance of these three groups varies, but in several countries, the mental and MSDs are two to four times more frequent than cardiovascular disorders as causes for disability pensions.

No country provides statistics for CMP as a medical cause for disability pensions. However, muscle pain/fibromyalgia is frequently used as a diagnosis on application schemes. In Norway, these conditions were the primary diagnoses for 18% of persons with disability pensions due to MSDs in 1997, second only to low back pain (44%), but more frequent than both rheumatoid arthritis (9%)

Table 1.2 Distribution (in percent) of persons on disability pensions due to musculoskeletal and connective tissue disorders by diagnosis and gender, Norway, 31 December 1997 (based on National Insurance Administration, 1998).

Diagnosis	Men N= 26 623	Women N= 54 034	Total N= 80 657
Low back disorders	59	36	44
Rheumatoid arthritis	6	10	9
Osteoarthritis	13	12	12
Muscle pain/fibromyalgia	7	24	18
Other MSDs	15	18	17
Sum	**100**	**100**	**100**

and osteoarthritis (12%). Muscle pain/fibromyalgia was the primary diagnosis for 24% of women and 7% for men (Table 1.2).

Risk factors in contraction of disabling musculoskeletal disorders

The association between high prevalence of disability and low social status, measured as income level, educational level or social class, is usually strong. Disabling MSDs are more frequent among unmarried persons, indicating that lack of social support might be a risk factor for the development of disability.

Musculoskeletal disability is frequently associated with physical stress at the workplace, such as heavy lifting, repetitive movements and work paced by a machine (Mäkelä et al., 1993). Psychosocial work stress, e.g. work monotony and tight time schedules, was also significantly associated with disability, but to a lesser degree.

Trends for disability

A study on cohort patterns in disability and disease in adults born 1915–59, based on the US National Health Interview Survey, found more disabling MSDs in cohorts born after World War II (Reynolds et al., 1998). We might anticipate higher rates of disability as these cohorts enter old age, compared with earlier cohorts. In the period 1986–93, the number of awards for Social Security disabled worker benefits grew by 37% in USA, and the share of MSDs increased from 18% to 21% of the beneficiaries (Ferron, 1995). In Norway, the annual number of new beneficiaries with disability pension has increased 36% in the period 1980–97. In addition, the proportion of disability pensions due to MSDs has increased, from 26% to 41% for women, and from 18% to 27% for men.

Thus, the prevalence of disabling MSDs seems to be increasing, while, as stated earlier, there are no firm indications that the prevalence of these disorders has increased in the population. If these findings can be confirmed, one must ask the intriguing question why this occurs. Have MDSs become more aggressive, causing more disability, or are the consequences increasingly difficult to live with in a more complex and demanding work environment?

The diagnosis of fibromyalgia has not been used consistently in any statistics for more than 10 years. The changes in sickness absence and disability pension rates that have been observed might be due to changes in the use of diagnoses. We need a longer time span with comparable observations before we can document time trends.

Utilization of healthcare services

Patients with MSDs are frequent visitors to primary healthcare centers, hospitals, and paramedical institutions (e.g. physiotherapy and chiropractic). In the Ontario Health Survey, they caused almost 20% of all healthcare utilization (Badley *et al.*, 1994).

There is little information on healthcare utilization by patients with CMP. Fibromyalgia patients have, however, high consultation rates with family physicians, high hospital admission rates, high rates of medication use (mostly analgesics) and very high rates for contact with other health professionals (Macfarlane *et al.*, 1999). Healthcare utilization in patients with fibromyalgia is comparable to patients with osteoarthritis and low back pain. Very high hospitalization rates have been noted prior to diagnosis of fibromyalgia, but dropped quickly thereafter (Cathey *et al.*, 1986).

There is a general impression that patients with musculoskeletal pain syndromes are becoming more frequent in family practice. A recent Swedish study showed that an increasing number of individuals with pain-related diagnoses consulted primary care physicians (from 156/1000 per year in 1987 to 193/1000 per year in 1996) (Andersson *et al.*, 1999). The increase was mainly due to patients with fibromyalgia or headache.

Healthcare costs

Healthcare costs generated by MSDs are stunning. In 1994, they constituted the second largest diagnostic group (after mental retardation) to generate healthcare costs in the Netherlands (Meerding *et al.*, 1998). The total direct cost for health services due to these disorders was 0.7% of the gross national budget. In studies from Canada and USA, the direct healthcare costs corresponded to 1.0% and 1.2% of gross national budgets respectively (Yelin and Callahan, 1996).

Direct healthcare costs include institution care, outpatient treatment and drug use (Meerding *et al.*, 1998), but disability also generates considerable indirect costs, i.e. lost productivity and wage loss. For MSDs, indirect costs appear to be greater than the direct costs, corresponding to 2.4% and 1.3% of the gross national budgets in Canada and USA.

Political issues

The question whether CMP should elicit welfare benefits or not has caused great controversy. After a period with frequent awards of disability claims in the 1970s, the US Social Security Administration (USSSA) terminated disability benefits for more than 500 000 persons in 1981–83. Chronic pain syndromes were over-represented among these terminations. This change in policy brought about numerous legal appeals and adverse publicity. Policy was again reversed, and 290 000 persons were reinstated as beneficiaries. Similar inconsistencies in disability benefit matters have occurred in other countries.

For the patients, such political ambiguity is clearly unsatisfactory. Their applications for social benefits are handled and decided upon in a seemingly haphazard and random manner. It might also appear as unjust that they are denied benefits, when persons with similar loss of function and work ability but with more acceptable diagnoses are granted benefits.

Due to the skewed sex distribution of CMP, the denials of benefits have had especially negative consequences for women. Denials have also been more frequent for persons with low levels of education (Claussen, 1998). Thus, the consequences of restricting disability benefits have struck different socioeconomic groups in an uneven way.

The increase of disability benefit applicants with CMP has been a problem for social security systems. Basically, the problem can be traced back to a dilemma in all modern welfare societies: how to balance the distribution of goods, according to work or according to needs. In most countries, certain needy groups, e.g. children, elderly and sick persons, are exempt from the general rule of working. Children and the elderly are easily defined by simple age limits, but the definition as to who is sick has caused continuous tension as the welfare systems have developed. The medical profession has been given the task to decide these matters.

To guide decisions, 'work disability due to disease or injury' has commonly been used as a criterion. Initially, this was interpreted as being recognizable impairment in bodily organs, i.e visible signs, laboratory tests or other 'objective' results from medical examination. However, disorders such as CMP cause disability without giving clear signs of organ impairment. In this situation, various means to ease the tension have been recommended. In a US report on 'pain and disability' (Osterweis *et al.*, 1987), it was suggested to focus more on work ability, and less on the underlying disease, illness or complaints. Thus, patients with chronic pain should be tested for functional level and work capacity as early as possible in the evaluation process. Benefit evaluation should seek evidence not only of underlying disease processes, but also consider serious functional limitations and other effects on the claimants' lives. A stronger focus on disability, rather than on the underlying disease, has been suggested also in other countries.

Conclusion

Musculoskeletal conditions as seen in epidemiological studies comprise a heterogeneous group of conditions with different etiology and different prognosis.

There is no simple continuum from short-term localized complaints to chronic widespread complaints. In the clinical setting we are able to diagnose some diseases with accepted criteria, such as rheumatoid arthritis and sciatica. Still, both in the population and among patients consulting family physicians or specialists we find a large group of persons with complaints we do not understand, and where the medical establishment disagrees as to what it is, and what to do with it.

The consequences of MSDs on function and work ability are profound in most countries, and cause substantial costs for the individual and for society. CMP has not been studied to the same extent, but appears to have considerable negative consequences for a large number of people. CMP is more frequent in women, increases by age and is associated with low status, manual labor, and physical and psychological stress at the workplace. The more associated symptoms, and the more widespread, the more observable is the female dominance. CMP has often been rejected as a reason for benefits, and continues to cause tension in the social benefit systems.

The big challenge is that chronic widespread musculoskeletal complaints have not really been taken seriously by clinicians or researchers. The hope is that this book will help healthcare practitioners better understand the health and social needs of CMP and CWP sufferers.

References

Aarflot T (1999) *Is chronic widespread musculoskeletal pain part of a multisymptom syndrome?* (dissertation). University of Oslo, Oslo, Norway. Unpublished.

Aarflot T and Bruusgaard D (1994) Chronic musculoskeletal complaints and subgroups with special reference to uric acid. *Scand J Rheumatol.* **23**(1): 25–9.

Andersson HI, Ejlertsson G, Leden I and Scherstén B (1999) Musculoskeletal chronic pain in general practice: studies of healthcare utilisation in comparison with pain prevalence. *Scand J Prim Health Care.* **17**: 87–92.

Badley EM, Rasooly I and Webster GK (1994) Relative importance of musculoskeletal disorders as a cause of chronic health problems, disability, and health care utilization: findings from the 1990 Ontario Health Survey. *J Rheumatol.* **21**: 505–14.

Barton N (1989) Repetitive strain disorder. *BMJ.* **299**: 405–6.

Bernhard BP (1997) *Musculoskeletal Disorders and Workplace Factors: a critical review of epidemiologic evidence for work-related musculoskeletal disorders of the neck, upper extremity, and low back.* Publication No. 97–141, US Department of Health and Human Services, Cincinnati, OH.

Brage S, Nygård JF and Tellnes G (1998) The gender gap in musculoskeletal-related long-term sickness absence in Norway. *Scand J Soc Med.* **26**: 34–43.

Bruusgaard D, Smedbraaten BK and Natvig B (2000) Bodily pain, sleep problems and mental distress in schoolchildren. *Acta Paediatr* **89**: 597–600.

Buskila D, Neumann L, Hershman E *et al.* (1995) Fibromyalgia syndrome in children: an outcome study. *J Rheumatol.* **22**(3): 525–8.

Cathey MA, Wolfe F, Kleinheksel SM and Hawley DJ (1986) Socioeconomic impact of fibrositis: a study of 81 patients with primary fibrositis. *Am J Med.* **81**: 78–84.

Claussen B (1998) Restricting the influx of disability beneficiaries by law: experiences in Norway. *Scand J Prim Health Care.* **26**: 1–7.

Clauw DJ and Chrousos GP (1997) Chronic pain and fatigue syndromes: overlapping clinical and neuroendocrine features and potential pathogenic mechanisms. *Neuroimmunomodulation.* **4**(3): 134–53.

Croft PR, Rigby AS, Boswell R, Schollum J and Silman AJ (1993) Prevalence of chronic widespread pain in the general population. *J Rheumatol.* **20**: 710–13.

Ferron DT (1995) Diagnostic trends of disabled social security beneficiaries, 1986–93. *Soc Secur Bull.* **58**: 15–31.

Kristjansdottir G (1997) Prevalence of pain combinations and overall pain: a study of headache, stomach pain and back pain among school children. *Scand J Soc Med.* **25**(1): 58–63.

Macfarlane GJ (1999) Fibromyalgia and chronic widespread pain. In: I Crombie, P Croft, S Linton *et al.* (eds) *Epidemiology of Pain.* IASP Press, Seattle, WA.

Macfarlane GJ, Croft PR, Schollum J and Silman AJ (1996) Widespread pain: is an improved classification possible? *J Rheumatol.* **23**: 1628–32.

Macfarlane GJ, Hunt IM, McBeth J, Papageorgiou AC and Silman AJ (1999) Chronic widespread pain in the community: influences on healthcare seeking behaviour. *J Rheumatol.* **26**: 413–19.

Mäkelä M, Heliövaara M, Sievers K *et al.* (1993) Musculoskeletal disorders as determinants of disability in Finns aged 30 years or more. *J Clin Epidemiol.* **46**: 549–59.

Meerding WJ, Bonneux L, Polder JJ, Koopmanschap MA and van der Maas PJ (1998) Demographic and epidemiological determinants of healthcare costs in Netherlands: cost of illness study. *BMJ.* **317**: 111–15.

Merskey H and Bogduk N (1994) *Classification of Chronic Pain.* IASP Press, Seattle, WA.

Mikkelsson M, Salminen JJ and Kautiainen H (1997) Non-specific musculoskeletal pain in pre-adolescents: prevalence and 1-year persistence. *Pain.* **73**(1): 29–35.

Natvig B, Nessioy I, Bruusgaard D and Rutle O (1994) Musculoskeletal complaints in a population: occurrence and localization. *Tidssk Nor Laegeforen.* **114**(3): 323–7.

Osterweis M, Kleinmann A and Mechanic D (eds) (1987) *Pain and Disability: clinical, behavioral, and public health perspectives.* National Academy Press, Washington DC.

Reynolds DL, Chambers LW, Badley EM *et al.* (1992) Physical disability among Canadians reporting musculoskeletal diseases. *J Rheumatol.* **19**: 1020–30.

Reynolds SL, Crimmins EM and Saito Y (1998) Cohort differences in disability and disease presence. *Gerontologist.* **38**: 578–90.

Shorter E (1995) Sucker-punched again!: physicians meet the disease of the month syndrome. *J Psychosom Med.* **39**: 115–18.

Smedbråten BK, Natvig B, Rutle O and Bruusgaard D (1998) Self-reported bodily pain in school children. *Scand J Rheumatol.* **27**: 273–6.

Smythe HA (1985) Fibrositis and other diffuse musculoskeletal syndromes. In: WN Kelly, ED Harris and S Russy (eds) *Textbook of Rheumatology.* WB Saunders, Philadelphia, PA.

Szubert Z, Sobala W and Zycinska Z (1997) The effect of system restructuring on absenteeism due to sickness in the work place (In Polish). *Med Pr.* **48**: 543–51.

Tellnes G, Svendsen K-O, Bruusgaard D and Bjerkedal T (1989) Incidence of sickness certification: proposal for use as a health status indicator. *Scand J Prim Health Care.* **7**: 111–17.

Ursin H (1997) Sensitization, somatization and subjective health complaints. *Int J Behav Med.* **4**: 105–16.

White KP, Speechley M, Harth M and Ostbye T (1999) Comparing self-reported function and work disability in 100 community cases of fibromyalgia syndrome versus controls in London, Ontario: the London fibromyalgia epidemiology study. *Arthritis Rheum.* **42**: 76–83.

Wolfe F, Smythe HA, Yunus MB *et al.* (1990) The American College of Rheumatology 1990 criteria for the classification of fibromyalgia. *Arthritis Rheum.* **33**(2): 160–72.

Yelin E and Callahan LF (1996) The economic cost and social and psychological impact of musculoskeletal conditions: National Arthritis Data Work Groups. *Arthritis Rheum.* **38**: 1351–62.

Yunus MB, Masi AT and Alday JC (1989) Preliminary criteria for primary fibromyalgia syndrome. *Clin Exp Rheumatol.* **21**: 63–9.

2

The disease: chronic myofascial pain

In the middle of the night, Judith Smith wakes up and feels terrible. Her body is aching, in a way that reminds her of the time she fell down the staircase and found herself lying black and blue, helpless on the floor. However, no specific accident has occurred for years, although minor strains certainly may happen when the workload and pace at work is high. Judith Smith watched a television show last week, dealing with nerves and muscles and other health and body stuff. Since then, she can clearly imagine how her blood vessels spread oxygen around her body. Still, she does not understand how muscles can be so sore and painful. The muscles on the television seemed so fresh and healthy. Her own muscle cells must be broken to pieces, or perhaps be out of order. She hopes her physician has a test to check and perhaps rule out this terrible suspicion of hers.

Muscle and pain physiology

Arne Tjølsen and Nina K Vøllestad

The sense of pain is a necessary part of the body's defence systems. Pain generally warns us when we are subject to stimuli that may cause tissue damage, either acutely or if the stimulus goes on over time. The ability to experience pain is therefore necessary for normal function during daily life. But although pain is necessary, in some instances it evolves into a long-lasting problem which seriously reduces the quality of life.

The IASP has defined pain like this:

An unpleasant sensory and emotional experience associated with actual or potential tissue damage, or described in terms of such damage.

Pain is an experience, which may be caused by tissue damage, but not necessarily so. The definition emphasizes the subjective experience of pain, and one of the most important consequences is that pain must be considered as real even if no disease or damage can be identified as the cause of the pain sensation.

The first well-formulated theory of how the perception of pain is modulated or regulated in the spinal cord was presented by Ronald Melzack and Patrick D Wall in 1965, and named the gate-control theory (Melzack and Wall, 1965). Since then it has been of considerable interest in the physiology of pain, and in its treatment.

This chapter outlines the parts of the nervous system involved in the sensation of pain, and describes those properties of the system which may cause changes in function and thereby cause long-lasting or chronic pain states.

From tissue to experience

When the body is exposed to a potentially harmful stimulus, a message is relayed from recording organs (receptors) in the tissue through several levels of neurones to the cerebral cortex and other areas of the brain. Such receptors, called nociceptors, are free nerve endings, and are found in most parts of the body. Nociceptors may respond to mechanical stimulation, such as pressure or stretch, to hot or cold and to chemical irritants in the tissue. The extent to which we will experience pain depends on a number of factors that regulate the sensitivity for pain. The nociceptors themselves may change sensitivity, so that they respond differently to the same stimulus over time. The conduction of the information through the spinal cord also may change, so that the central nervous system (CNS) responds more (or less) strongly to the stimulus, and the experience of pain hence becomes different.

Nociceptors are typical in that they can increase their sensitivity when the surrounding tissue is damaged. This increased sensitivity is caused by changes

---

Box 2.1   *Factors in the tissue contributing to increased sensitivity to pain*

- Histamine
- Serotonin
- Bradykinin
- ATP
- Neurokinins, e.g. substance P
- pH (protons)
- Potassium ions

in the environment of the nociceptors in and near damaged tissue and the release of a number of substances that contribute to the increased nociceptive sensitivity (Box 2.1). Many of these substances contribute to the development of an inflammatory response.

The central nervous system

Important relay stations for nociceptive signals from the tissues to the cerebral cortex are located in the dorsal horn of the spinal cord, in the brain stem and in the thalamus (Figure 2.1). Here there are synapses between the neurones, and it is in the areas with synapses that the signals may be modulated. In this way, what is passed on is dependent on the state of the nervous system. The

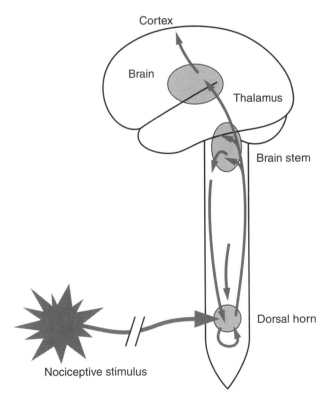

Figure 2.1 Schematic overview of the nociceptive pathways from peripheral tissue to the cerebral cortex. The signals travel through the spinal cord, the brain stem and the thalamus. At these sites the transmission of pain information can be changed. In the spinal cord, the pain signals are modulated by activity in local interneurones, by signals from other segments of the spinal cord, and by signals in nerve pathways from the brain stem.

information that reaches the cerebral cortex and that we experience consciously as pain is not exactly related to the cause of pain, but is influenced by the modulatory systems. This influence may be considerable.

The modulating systems in the spinal cord, working together with areas of the brain stem, are very important components in the ability of the nervous system to change its sensitivity to nociceptive stimulation. A network of nerve cells gives the possibility of change and adaptation of the nociceptive signals. A segment of the spinal cord that conveys information on pain also receives signals from other stimuli, both from the same body area and from other parts of the body. The spinal cord also receives signals from the brain and the brain stem (Figure 2.2). All these signals modulate the extent to which information about pain is forwarded to the cerebral cortex.

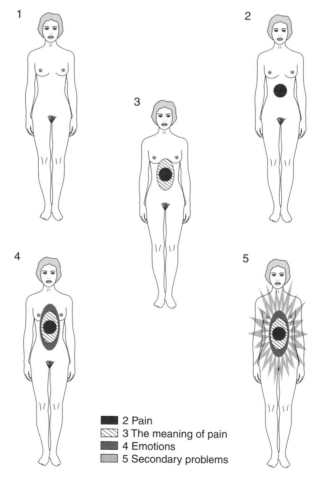

2 Pain
3 The meaning of pain
4 Emotions
5 Secondary problems

Figure 2.2 The components of the pain experience.

Muscle: a pathologic link?

Patients suffering from pain often describe muscle as the site(s) of pain. In particular, chronic pain is frequently located in muscles in the neck and shoulder region. Yet, the underlying muscular mechanisms are still debated. Several authors have argued that processes in the muscle may serve as pathogenetic links between several etiological causes of pain (e.g. psychic stress or monotonous work) and the individual experience of pain. The basis for such an understanding is given below.

There is much evidence of an association between workload and chronic musculoskeletal pain. Support for this has come from epidemiological studies, showing heavy workloads, repetitive and monotonous work and psychological stress to be risk factors for the cause of pain (Bongers et al., 1993; Hagberg et al., 1995). In addition, experimental studies show that pain may increase during work (Brox et al., 1997). Of particular interest is the observation that when pain is already present, the work-induced pain is enhanced. These observations indicate that processes connected to muscle activation and work can initiate pain or modulate already existing experience of pain.

It is well established that mechanical work and psychological load both may lead to increased muscle activation, even in muscles without an obvious functional demand for activation. An understanding of how muscle activation can influence nociceptors could, therefore, be of importance in finding common ground regarding the patient's situation and the management.

Muscles are composed of muscle fibers, each of which is innervated by one motor nerve. One nerve cell connects to several muscle fibers, and the unit comprising the motor nerve and all the muscle fibers it innervates is called a motor unit. The nociceptors are located between the muscle fibers and particularly between the tendon filaments at the ends of the muscle and along the blood vessels. Any factors inducing altered activation of nociceptors must therefore have an effect outside the muscle cells. The nociceptors cannot sense what occurs inside the cells, since they are basically located between the cells in muscle and tendon. We will, therefore, focus on changes that might act on these free nerve endings as a response to muscle activation.

When a motoneurone is activated, either voluntarily or involuntarily, all the muscle fibers in a motor unit are activated simultaneously and the muscle fibers contract. One consequence of this pattern is that, most often, some muscle fibers are active while others are at rest. A pressure is generated by the contracting muscle fibers, and hence the nociceptors are exposed to altering mechanical pressure. In addition, the shear forces developed between active and inactive muscle fibers may enhance the response of the nociceptors.

Precise control of muscle tension is important for normal functioning, and is achieved through an extensive interaction between various inputs to the motoneurones from several levels in the central and peripheral nervous system. At the motoneurone pool level, tension can be altered by varying the number of active motor units (recruitment) and by varying the firing rate and pattern in each motor unit (rate coding). Since muscle pain can be developed in muscles mainly generating low force contractions (e.g. less than 5% of the maximal force), activation of large proportions of the muscle is not required for development of symptoms (Hagberg *et al.*, 1995). The cause of pain could be related to sustained or repeated activation of a few motor units only.

Muscular processes during work

When a muscle is activated, action potentials are propagated across the muscle fibers, and this results in release of potassium ions into the extracellular fluid. This release will, within a few minutes, be balanced by an increased reuptake, and the extracellular accumulation levels off. As long as the activation is sustained, an elevated potassium concentration is seen in the interstitial fluid even at relatively low activation levels (Sejersted and Vøllestad, 1993).

When an adequate amount of oxygen is provided by the arterial blood, the energy release during muscle work can be fully oxidative. In this situation, the metabolic products are eliminated by the venous effluent blood. However, inadequate blood supply is often seen. One situation which may lead to this is when the energy demand exceeds the cardiovascular capacity for oxygen supply. An example of such a situation is intense exercise (e.g. running) which can be sustained for only a few minutes. Occlusion of the blood vessels can also lead to inadequate oxygen supply. This may occur when muscle contractions are sustained, and the pressure developed exceeds the perfusion pressure. For some muscles, occlusion may occur at force levels below 20% of maximal force (Sejersted and Vøllestad, 1993). Thus, anaerobic energy release may occur even during low-level exercise. If the blood supply is inadequate, large metabolic changes occur inside the muscle fibers, and these changes lead to changes also in the extracellular fluid. One of the most prominent metabolic changes is an accumulation of lactic acid, which will result in reduced pH. Even though such metabolic changes may influence nociceptors, it is still unclear whether they are of any importance for development of chronic pain.

It is well known that sympathetic nerves are brought into play simultaneously with activation of motoneurones. Noradrenaline is released in the muscles and adrenaline is released into the blood stream from the adrenal medulla. The sympathetic nervous activity and the catecholamine release are shown to depend both on the intensity and the duration of the muscle activation. The higher the muscle force (degree of activation), the larger is the response of the sympathetic system (Kjær *et al.*, 1987). During moderate, but constant, exercise levels, a gradual rise in sympathetic activation is reported. Hence, prolonged muscle activation will provide a gradually stronger stimulus for the nociceptors. The level of noradrenaline in venous blood indicates that the concentration in muscle tissue may well contribute to stimulation or sensitization of nociceptors. Other agents released during muscle activation may also stimulate the nociceptors.

A few studies have been conducted to compare the sympathetic nervous activity during exercise in patients having widespread pain such as fibromyalgia, and healthy subjects. The exercise regimen has been both sustained contraction for only a few minutes, and repetitive isometric contractions for a prolonged period of time. The sympathetic nervous activity recorded during shorter, sustained contractions was comparable in patients and healthy subjects. During prolonged exercise, however, blood samples indicated an attenuated release of adrenaline and noradrenaline in patients compared with healthy subjects. If these observations reflect a general phenomenon, pain is not closely related to increased sympathetic nervous activity.

As documented above, nociceptors located in muscle receive ample possible stimulators during normal muscle activation. Yet, in healthy humans only marginal increases in pain are experienced during exercise of various kinds (Brox et al., 1997). There is thus reason to believe that this nociceptive input to the CNS normally does not cause further activation of nociceptive pathways, which may be due to a physiological, ongoing endogenous inhibition of nociceptive signals. In contrast, when patients having chronic musculoskeletal pain perform similar types of exercise, the increase in pain is pronounced. For instance, patients with chronic rotator tendinosis or neck/shoulder myalgia reported a pain increase to almost 50% of maximal tolerable pain during two to three minutes' sustained low-force contraction of the shoulder muscles. It is, furthermore, interesting to note that in patients with a unilateral affliction, the pain also increased markedly at the non-afflicted side. These observations suggest that the input from muscle through the nociceptors is altered by the presence of even moderate pain. Furthermore, pain is clearly evoked by muscle activation, but only by patients already experiencing pain.

Prolonged and repeated work bouts

It is well established that work involving sustained or repetitive work, often of quite monotonous character, is a risk factor for developing chronic musculoskeletal pain (Bongers et al., 1993; Hagberg et al., 1995). This observation has prompted the hypothesis that prolonged activation or repeated activation of the same muscles for a long time induces changes which eventually evoke pain. Several mechanisms have been proposed as important, among which muscle fatigue, loss of muscle cell integrity, altered electrolyte balance (potassium and calcium) and lack of energy substrates have been mostly discussed.

Most of the processes occurring in muscles during work are normalized within a short time if the muscle is allowed to rest, and the blood supply is not occluded. After long-lasting, low-level work, most changes will be reversed by a good night's sleep. For instance, energy substrates such as muscular glycogen are utilized and may be completely exhausted during exercise. After 24 hours or less, normal resting values are again attained. Some authors have observed a small fraction of muscle fibers with almost no ATP and they interpreted this as a response to repeated and sustained muscle activation, a sort of 'overload'. Experimental studies have, however, been unable to provide firm evidence in support of this hypothesis.

Some changes may prevail or continue to change after the end of work. One muscular factor that seems to have a slow recovery after prolonged activation is the depressed force generating capacity. This response, often called muscular fatigue, is rapidly reversed after short-lasting, intense exercise, resulting in almost complete recovery within minutes of rest. In other situations, when fatigue is developed more slowly, only marginal recovery is seen over the first 30–60 minutes of rest. When the same type of work is repeated day after day, the recovery process may not have time to operate fully between bouts. It should also be emphasized that in today's society, there is little difference between the type of muscle work at home and at work. Hence, the time for recovery processes in muscles might be even shorter outside the work place.

The experience of pain is often related to fatigue (Russel, 1996). Experimental studies have shown, at least for pain patients, that fatigue and pain may develop in parallel. Several possible mechanisms for an association between fatigue and pain have been proposed, but firm evidence is still lacking. On the other hand, substantial fatigue may occur in healthy persons without any experience of pain (Brox *et al.*, 1997). Hence, there is no universal relationship between these two phenomena.

Little attention has been paid to mechanical mechanisms as a possible contributor to development of symptoms. Due to the hierarchical order of recruitment, two neighboring muscle fibers may have quite different activation levels, and thus have a different mechanical behavior. For instance, during light manual work or cognitively demanding tasks, only a small proportion of the muscle fibers in the trapezius muscle is active. The active motor units are activated at subtetanic levels, meaning that the force they develop is not fused. Rather, the active muscle fibers show an oscillating behavior. During repetitive contractions, it is shown that the amplitude of these oscillations increases progressively (Vøllestad *et al.*, 1997). This temporal pattern is caused by a gradual increase in relaxation rate. One consequence of this response is that the nociceptors located between the muscle fibers or in the tendon are exposed to a continuous mechanical strain, which increases with duration of muscle activation. It should also be mentioned that the increases in relaxation rate and oscillation amplitude show a very slow recovery. Hence, incomplete recovery between work bouts could contribute to changes over time. In addition, exercise may induce processes not necessarily reflected during the contractions, but rather developed more slowly over the next couple of days.

The link between these mechanical factors, nociception and pain experience remains unclear. It is not known whether the nociceptors adapt over time with repeated stimulation and reduce the signal transmission to the CNS. The observation that patients suffering from chronic pain tend to respond with a much larger increase in pain during work than healthy persons suggests that there is no adaptation. Rather, the opposite is indicated.

In conclusion, there are several possibilities for muscle to serve as a pathogenetic link between physical work or mental loads and development of musculoskeletal pain. We are not yet able to point out clearly the responsible mechanisms. It should also be emphasised that so far there is little evidence of muscles with chronic pain responding differently from normal healthy muscles to a single contraction or exercise bout. However, the responses and stimuli generated by muscles are apparently interpreted differently by the CNS when pain is present.

Acute pain

The perception of an acutely painful stimulus varies between individuals, and in one person it is context dependent. Locally in the spinal cord there are nerve cells with short axons, which inhibit the transfer of nociceptive information. These may have morphine-like substances (e.g. enkephalins) or smaller molecules as transmitters. Long pathways from nerve cells in the brain stem may also influence the signal transmission. These long pathways may generally inhibit the pain sensitivity as well.

In these mechanisms, we find part of the explanation to common phenomena when the perception of pain varies with time and context. It is common to assume that non-painful stimulation close to a painful area may stimulate pain-attenuating mechanisms locally in the spinal network of nerve cells. This leads to a reduction of pain perception. Massage, manipulation and some forms of transcutaneous electrical nerve stimulation (TENS) may work through such mechanisms. In addition, it seems that stronger stimulation that activates nociceptors also gives an attenuated sensitivity for pain from other parts of the body (Le Bars *et al.*, 1979). This phenomenon is caused by painful stimulation activating areas in the brain stem, which may inhibit the transmission of nociceptive information at the spinal level through long descending pathways.

Treatment of pain with acupuncture and some forms of TENS probably works partly by activation of these systems.

In addition to the sensitization of nociceptors in peripheral tissue, the sensitivity to nociceptive information may also increase in the spinal cord and in the brain. During and after strong nociceptive stimulation the spinal cord will have increased sensitivity, and weaker stimulation may elicit pain. These phenomena in the CNS are included in the term 'central sensitization'. Mechanisms both peripherally in the tissues and in the CNS may lead to a spread of sensitization, so that the greater sensitivity to pain is increased outside the area that initially was exposed to noxious stimulation. It is characteristic of the central sensitization that the increase of area is considerably larger than the increase due to peripheral sensitization (Coderre *et al.*, 1993).

Chronic pain and long-time sensitization of the nervous system

The modulation of long-lasting pain and the mechanisms of development of chronic pain are considerably less known than the modulation of acute pain. Why does pain sometimes continue for a long time although the original cause has been removed or has disappeared? It is probable that there are long-lasting changes in the spinal pain modulating systems so that their function is altered. This may lead to an unwanted increase in pain sensitivity, and thereby to pain which is not directly caused by a peripheral noxious stimulus, but by altered function in the CNS (Coderre *et al.*, 1993).

How do the nerve cells change?

Strong noxious stimulation is a factor that may elicit such a change of function in the spinal cord. In experiments on animals in general anesthesia it is found that nerve cells in the spinal cord change their function during strong stimulation, so that repeated stimulation of nociceptors induces an increased transmission of nociceptive information, and an increased nerve cell response. It is characteristic of this effect that the increased pain transmission is caused only by stimulation of nociceptive nerve fibres (Cook *et al.*, 1987). With this kind of stimulation, the response to noxious stimulation is increased, but not the response to touch or other non-painful stimulation.

Pain stimulation may also cause spinal nerve cells to respond to stimulation of a larger area. These changes may be considerable (Cook *et al.*, 1987). A nerve cell that initially responds to stimulation of a limited area may begin to react to stimulation quite far from the original area. It seems that this increase of response is particularly strong after stimulation of deep tissues, such as muscle (Wall and Woolf, 1984). Nerve cells that only respond to strong, potentially painful stimulation may also begin to respond to weaker stimulation, such as touch (Willis, 1993). In several pathological pain states this is just the case: stimulation that normally will not be considered painful is perceived as pain. This makes these findings particularly interesting, because the mechanisms may be similar to what happens in patients in pain.

The major transmitter that is released in the spinal cord from sensory nerve cells is glutamate. This is also true for cells connected to nociceptors. It turns out that glutamate may cause relatively long-lasting stimulation of nociceptive cells in the spinal cord, by binding to certain receptors (called NMDA receptors). In addition, such a stimulation produces a number of changes in the metabolism that may cause long-lasting changes in the sensitivity of the nerve cells.

Inhibition of this glutamate effect will attenuate the increase of pain sensitivity after strong, painful stimulation (Svendsen *et al.*, 1998). If local anesthesia, glutamate inhibitors or opioids are given after the onset of pain, the effect on pain is considerably weaker. This indicates that the cause of the increased sensitivity is the acute pain, and that the effect of glutamate on the NMDA receptors in the spinal cord is important. The sensitivity may be increased for several hours after pain stimulation. In experiments, it has been shown that inhibition of the NMDA receptors may attenuate the development of pain states after nerve damage or neuropathic pains.

Some sort of learning in the spinal cord seems to be of importance for the sensitivity to pain. The spinal pain systems may change their function and adapt to new situations by altering the processing of nociceptive signals, and sometimes this change causes more of the information to be interpreted as pain. This change of function as a response to stimulation is similar to learning processes, and it is likely that such processes in the spinal pain systems share some mechanisms with learning in the brain.

In addition to glutamate, neuropeptides, e.g. substance P, are released from nerve cells receiving signals from nociceptors. Neuropeptides are released more slowly than glutamate, and have more prolonged effects. Peptides act together with glutamate in pain transmission, so that a combined release may enhance the response. The release of peptides probably increases over time during persisting or repeated pain stimulation, which also increases pain perception.

Pain that lasts for some time, e.g. after tissue damage or inflammation, also causes a number of other changes in the CNS that may be associated with long-lasting functional changes (Coderre *et al.*, 1993). It is probable that changes in gene transcription and protein synthesis may be involved. It seems that an increased protein synthesis is caused by stimulation of the NMDA receptors, and may be reduced by both NMDA receptor antagonists and morphine.

Clinical evidence

Clinical experience and investigations in humans suggest that painful stimulation may cause long-lasting changes in the function of the CNS, and contribute to an increased pain sensitivity. It has been shown that pain after surgery may be reduced if the influx of nociceptive signals to the spinal cord during surgery is minimized (Ejlertsen *et al.*, 1992). Several studies indicate that effective block of the nociceptive signals by local anesthesia, regional blocks or spinal/epidural anesthesia before they reach the CNS may reduce post-surgical pain. The application of anesthetic techniques to reduce nociceptive activation during surgical procedures has been termed 'pre-emptive analgesia'. A number of clinical studies have been performed indicating that this actually is clinically important in reducing long-lasting pain after surgery (Kato *et al.*, 2000; Katz *et al.*, 1992).

When pain becomes long-lasting

There is now experimental evidence of the ability of the nociceptive systems to change their functions for long periods of time. The changes in the peripheral tissues where pain often originates are quite well known, and we know that the receptors that respond to noxious stimulation may increase their sensitivity considerably. The response to the nociceptive signals in the CNS varies, and we know that the spinal regulatory mechanisms can, in some cases, cause a long-term increase in the sensitivity for pain.

The peripheral and central mechanisms may influence each other, and with long-lasting pain a positive feedback loop may develop, enhancing the pain (Ursin *et al.*, 1993). It has been suggested that increased nociceptor activity may lead to increased activation of motoneurones. By this mechanism, increased muscle activation at rest is also predicted, which again may increase nociceptor activity. The existence of such a vicious circle is still debated. The increased pain perception in pain patients during muscular work suggests an increased sensitivity either of nociceptors or in more central pathways of pain perception. Nociceptive signals to the CNS may also cause reflexes in the autonomous nervous system, with an increased sympathetic activity, and this is also likely to increase the nociceptor sensitivity.

At the same time, the ongoing nociceptive stimulation will cause an increased sensitivity for nociceptive signals also in the CNS, and this will be a crucial component in the positive feedback loop enhancing the pain.

We have a considerable amount of knowledge of how pain itself can lead to an increase in pain sensitivity in the spinal cord, and also some knowledge of which mechanisms are involved in these processes. It is likely that pain conditions with a variety of causes may give overstimulation of other parts of the CNS, as well as of the spinal cord, with the associated risk of long-lasting function changes. If this is the case, the consequence will have to be that pain of a significant strength and duration should be treated actively and sufficiently.

Most hypotheses for long-lasting changes in pain sensitivity assume an episode of strong noxious stimulation that has triggered the changes. However, it is clear that long-lasting and chronic pain conditions with enhanced pain sensitivity may occur without an identifiable episode of acute, nociceptive pain in the patient's history. In such cases, the mechanisms may be similar to those triggered by noxious stimulation. It is possible that long-term changes may be caused by different kinds of hyperactivity in the CNS. Mechanisms resembling cellular learning and memory, which increase the responsiveness of neurones in local areas of the neuronal network, are possible in such a development. It is also likely that feedback loops may originate more gradually, where there is reciprocal stimulation of the peripheral and central nociceptive systems. Thus, a situation with long-lasting pain may develop without a single episode of strong, acute pain starting the process.

Pain is a complex experience that affects the whole individual, and that influences and is influenced by psychological states. An understanding of psychological factors involved in the patient's suffering is essential for good pain treatment. Our understanding is, however, that the sensation and experience of pain is always based on real, physiological processes in the nervous system. The patient's personal experiences and social and psychological factors all contribute to modulate the function of the nervous system. The way nociceptive information is handled on its way to or within the brain will, in the end, determine how pain is felt and experienced by each individual.

Prevailing multidimensional models for clinical understanding of chronic pain syndromes

Rae Frances Bell

Until the early 1960s the current theory of pain generation and pain experience was unidimensional. This 'biomedical' model considered pain as a purely sensory–physical experience where identification of the somatic cause would ultimately result in treatment and resolution of the pain. If no somatic cause was identified, the problem was labelled 'psychogenic'. This approach has its roots in the Cartesian mind–body dualism, whereby body and psyche are considered to be totally separate entities. The biomedical approach to chronic nonmalignant pain proved ultimately to be fruitless.

Melzack and Wall's gate-control theory was an attempt to integrate neurophysiological findings and the influence of psychological processes on pain perception and response into a comprehensive theory of pain. Fordyce (1976) later proposed a behavioral theory of pain, drawing attention to the importance of environmental feedback on behavior, specifically pain behavior. These theories have today led to the recognition that pain is a perceptual experience, a complex, multidimensional phenomenon. The current biopsychosocial pain model which will be presented in this chapter enables a better clinical understanding of chronic, non-malignant pain. This model, however, still fails to provide an explicit explanation for the inter-relation of sensory–physical and emotional aspects of pain. Recently, Melzack (1999) has proposed an explanation for this inter-relation where affective, behavioral, cognitive and sensory–physical facets are envisioned as an overarching, integrated chronic pain system.

What causes chronic pain?

Despite considerable advances in pain research and treatment, the exact mechanisms involved in the development and maintenance of chronic pain are still largely unknown from a clinical point of view. The pain stimulus may be due to persistent or recurrent nociception, e.g. in the case of a patient with rheumatoid arthritis, having frequent inflammatory joint affection, or a patient with osteoporosis having compression fractures of the vertebrae and secondary muscle pain. However, in the large majority of chronic pain patients it is difficult to identify a nociceptive stimulus. In most cases, the pain may have originally arisen in response to injury, but persists long after healing, i.e. after the nociceptive stimulus has disappeared.

The pain stimulus may also be due to dysfunction in the nervous system, due to permanent nervous tissue damage: damage to the peripheral or CNS may give rise to persistent and troublesome neuropathic pain, as in phantom pain, post-stroke pain and post-herpetic neuralgia.

Box 2.2   *Factors associated with pain intensity*

- Cognitive factors
- Attentional focus
- The meaning of the pain
- Circumstances surrounding the pain
- Learning and prior experience
- Emotions
- Self-efficacy

From a clinical point of view, it is perhaps more constructive to pose the questions, what causes pain to persist and what makes the pain so painful? It is now generally recognized that pain intensity is not directly related to the physical pathology causing the pain. The intensity of pain and the responses to perception of pain are influenced by a wide range of factors, including attentional focus, the meaning of the pain, prior learning, prior experience and others shown in Box 2.2 (Turk, 1996).

Cognitive factors

Pain is a signal of tissue damage or impending damage. Pain signals are interpreted, and, dependent on the interpretation, may be experienced as more or less painful. A number of studies have demonstrated that patients' beliefs, attitudes and expectancies influence both their reports of pain (Turk, 1996) and their response to treatment. Even the way we think about pain seems to influence how painful it is. For example, 'catastrophizing' is a style of thinking anticipating extremely negative outcomes of an experience (such as a pain). Catastrophizing is a so-called 'cognitive error' which appears to significantly influence pain and disability (Turk, 1996).

Attentional focus

Pain signals demand our attention. When we understand the cause of the pain, and are sure that the pain does not signal danger, we can 'let go' of the pain. There is no longer a need to focus on these particular sensory signals. In the case of chronic pain, the pain has lost its danger-signal value. Chronic pain patients are often unsure of the exact cause of the pain, are afraid that the pain may signal danger or damage and focus constantly on these sensory signals. Pain 'catastrophizers' appear to be hypervigilant for threatening somatic information (Crombez et al., 1998). That is, they have trouble diverting attention from the pain. Diverting attention from the pain appears to relieve it (McCaul and Malott, 1984) and is the background for pain treatment involving teaching the patient to focus on other stimuli (attention-based cognitive coping strategies).

The meaning of the pain

When pain arises, our first reaction is to interpret the cause. The pain may be explainable and unthreatening, such as when we jam a finger in the door.

We know immediately the reason for the pain, and that this type of pain usually resolves. We then no longer need to bother about the pain, or to focus on the injury. However, the situation is quite different if the pain arises for no obvious reason, e.g. a back pain unrelated to strain/injury. Many chronic low back pain patients have been extensively examined within the healthcare system. They have listened carefully to all advice and evaluations, but lack the medical background to select which information is useful. A patient hearing that his or her back is 'hypermobile' may interpret this as a potentially dangerous situation, and thereafter becomes reluctant to move his or her back. A patient with a stomach-ache may first attribute this to food ('That garlic sausage I ate yesterday'). However, if the pain persists, the patient may adopt more alarming explanations such as malignancy ('Didn't Mother's bowel cancer start with a pain in the stomach?'). A woman with pain in the right groin, which radiates to the right hypochondrium when she lays down, despite her physician's reassurance, is convinced that the surgeon forgot an instrument in her abdomen. The character and localization of the pain cements her belief in the forgotten instrument, while her fear of the pain and the potential damage being done intensifies the pain. In the case of the chronic pain patient, the fact that extensive investigation has not uncovered pathology only exacerbates the situation ('It's so painful, there *must* be something drastically wrong, and doctors are always missing cancer diagnoses'). Patients usually have their own private theories regarding the cause of the pain. The clinician, therefore, needs to elucidate this in order to correct misapprehensions which may be amplifying the pain or affecting the patient's behavior in such a way as to cause more (secondary) pain. It is usually not enough to point out that no alarming pathology has been discovered. The patient needs an (unalarming) explanation of the pain in order to be able to stop focusing on it.

Circumstances surrounding the pain

Not only the pain itself, but also the situation in which the pain occurs influences the intensity of the pain experienced. Chronic pain patients commonly report that the pain increases when they are in large gatherings or are stressed, and diminishes when they are enjoying themselves or absorbed in meaningful activity.

Learning and prior experience

From early childhood, we are conditioned to respond to pain in a specific manner. Some parents minimize painful incidents, whilst others make a fuss over the tiniest injury. The child, in turn, may learn to ignore or over-respond to painful stimuli. Prior experience may also be expected to influence the pain patient's coping strategies. There appears to be a relationship between traumatic events in childhood, such as physical and/or sexual abuse, and chronic pain later in life (Goldberg *et al.*, 1999). The child with trauma history does not develop adequate coping mechanisms to confront new illnesses or accidents in life. Any new trauma will exacerbate the patient's feeling of victimhood and helplessness.

Emotions

Anxiety may be likened to the volume control on the stereo player. Anxiety generally increases and maintains pain, whilst strategies ensuring a sense of security may diminish it. Recent studies (Crombez *et al.*, 1999) suggest that pain-related fear may be more disabling than pain itself. Many chronic pain patients are hostile and angry, especially towards healthcare workers and the social security system. These feelings of anger and frustration may compound treatment designed to alleviate the pain, by hindering patient motivation and increasing autonomic arousal (Fernandez and Turk, 1995). A large number of chronic pain patients are clinically depressed, most often as a consequence of the pain. Chronic pain patients commonly report disturbed sleep patterns. It is interesting to note that depression, pain and sleep share a common neurotransmitter, serotonin. Drugs used in the treatment of depression, principally the tricyclic antidepressants, have been demonstrated to relieve chronic pain.

Self-efficacy

The concept of self-efficacy is useful for understanding the chronic pain patient's pain. Most patients presenting to pain clinics feel helpless, and have no experience of being able to influence or control the pain. A large number of studies have shown that perceived self-efficacy is an important cognitive factor in controlling pain (Turk, 1996).

Chronification

Many of the discussed factors amplifying pain may also be involved in the chronification of pain. For example, pain 'catastrophizers' are traditionally unable to divert thought from the pain whilst anxiety and fear of pain may cause a hypervigilance, involving constant pain focus. Other possible factors involved in chronification of pain are inappropriate treatment modalities and dysfunctional coping.

Treatment

Repeated surgery, immobilization and inappropriate drugs may aggravate the pain. Many patients experience only partial pain relief with analgesics, at the same time reporting all the common side effects (tired, listless, headache, constipated, sleep disturbance). The medication may also be draining the patient's economic resources. Endless investigations and passive treatment modalities may indirectly serve to consolidate the patient's 'sick and helpless' role and thus contribute to chronification.

'Dysfunctional' coping

The strategy chosen by the patient to cope with the pain may ultimately increase and maintain the pain. By avoiding the pain, the patient may assume elaborate and unfortunate postures and ways of moving which give rise to new muscular or joint pain which, in turn, may be interpreted as an increase in the original pain ('They say there's nothing wrong with me, but it's getting worse all the time'). Drastically reducing physical activity and resting most of the day actually gives rise to a 'physical deconditioning syndrome' (Bortz, 1984) which can negatively affect both the emotional well-being and self-esteem of the patient. The patient has no perceived control over the pain, apart from taking analgesics, which are often ineffective, as mentioned above. The lack of effect of even strong analgesics, such as opioids, may be interpreted by the patient as evidence of the serious nature of the pain.

   Most chronic pain patients withdraw, have little social contact and are no longer engaged in meaningful activity. Family relations may be strained. The constant search for the *cause* of the pain ensures constant and unremitting focus.

The biopsychosocial model of chronic non-malignant pain

Even though we still have incomplete knowledge of the underlying mechanisms, the key to understanding chronic pain is that pain is a subjective experience, and that the perception of pain is influenced by a large number of factors, some of which are described above.

The biopsychosocial model focuses on the complex interaction of biological, psychological and social factors contributing to the individual patient's experience of pain and disability. Each patient must be evaluated individually, in order to identify the particular components of the pain experience.

Box 2.3 *The biopsychosocial model of pain*

The following is an illustration of how the biopsychosocial pain model may be used to understand a particular chronic pain problem. Mrs Smith's history has been incorporated as a clinical example.

The person

The individual having the pain may have had a normal, stable childhood environment and a relatively successful, uneventful adult life. Alternatively, the person having the pain may have been subjected to repeated abuse and trauma from an early age.

Mrs Judith Smith was one of five children. Her father was an alcoholic who regularly beat her two brothers and her mother. She has never mentioned this to her family physician.

The pain

In many patients the original pain focus may have disappeared and secondary pain is predominant when the pain has become chronic.

The meaning of the pain

As mentioned above, the patient's initial response is to try and understand the cause of the pain. Some patients seem unable to let go of frightening explanations, even when the physician reassures them. One example of this was a young woman with low back pain. At some stage during extensive investigation a doctor had said 'Your back may be a little unstable'. Even though no pathology could be identified, the young woman was convinced, and continued to be convinced, that 'Something is loose in my back'.

Mrs Judith Smith is worried about her chest pain. Her mother died of a heart attack, and she has read in a women's magazine that heart disease is often hereditary. In addition, she is worried about the pain in her shoulders and feet. Her family physician has told her that it's just muscular pain, but it's getting worse, and she's afraid she won't manage her job in the hospital laundry much longer.

Emotions concerning the pain

Depending on the patient's understanding of the pain, a number of emotions may arise. The patient who fears cancer will also fear the pain. The young woman who believes her back is 'loose' will also fear the pain and begin to do anything to avoid it. The woman who believes there is a pair of surgical scissors moving around amongst her intestines may become increasingly anxious. Fear and anxiety increase the intensity of the perceived pain, and make it difficult for the patient to focus thoughts away from the pain. As mentioned above, this fear of pain, or of incurring injury, may be more disabling than the pain itself.

In fact, Mrs Smith is quite anxious about the chest pain, though she hasn't said this to anyone. She has a friend whose husband has had two heart attacks. He can't exercise too much and her friend has to do all the heavy work. Mrs Smith is wondering whether the heavy work at the laundry could be affecting her heart.

Secondary factors contributing to the pain

Reduced physical activity

The patient commonly misinterprets the pain as being a 'danger signal'. This leads to avoidance behavior which may result in exaggerated resting, e.g. lying still for up to 20 hours a day. This in turn leads to rapid physical deconditioning. The patient may also adopt strange postures in order to avoid the pain. For example, the young woman with low back pain takes to walking bent forward, in order to avoid the pain. A few days of this strategy, and the result is increasing pain up the spine, radiating to neck and shoulders. This is intepreted by the patient to be an exacerbation of her back pain: 'They can't find anything wrong, but it's just getting worse and worse'.

Mrs Smith has stopped her evening walks. She's very tired and everything hurts. She has taken to spending the evening in a reclining chair, as she feels her heart 'needs a rest'. Her brother-in-law has lent her a pair of crutches, to help her poor feet. She only uses them in the house and it seemed to help a bit in the beginning, but now her shoulders are really playing up.

Treatment

The most common treatment pain patients receive is analgesic medication, often weak or stronger opioids. Some patients may experience relief of the pain and exhibit better function. However, many experience only partial or no pain relief, at the same time experiencing all the side effects such as drowsiness, lack of energy, headache, sleep disturbance and constipation. The young woman with back pain who believes she has a 'loose' back has now been operated on five times with spinal fusion at different levels. Following each operation, the pain just moves further up her spine. She is now using opioids, sometimes in injection form. She is spending most of the day lying down. Analgesic medication may actually sabotage attempts at rehabilitation, by giving insufficient relief and by draining energy which is needed to increase physical activity and for coping with the pain.

Mrs Smith has been using analgesics for years. First she had anti-inflammatory drugs, but she had trouble with her stomach. Then she was prescribed a muscle relaxant which seemed to help in the beginning, but after a while she had to take two tablets instead of one, as the pain was just increasing from week to week. Her family physician said she should not use so many muscle relaxants, so she tried to do without, but felt dreadful without them. The family physician then sighed and prescribed paracetamol–codeine, which worked quite well for a while. Then the pain was getting worse, and she had to increase the number of tablets. The family physician became quite annoyed and said she had to cut down. Mrs Smith went for two days without a single tablet, but the pain was dreadful, she felt unwell and could not sleep and just had to start again. Now she uses six tablets a day, the family physician will not let her have any more. It helps, just a little, so that she can relax a bit. But it doesn't really take away the pain. And if only she could sleep; she sleeps so badly, and never feels that she has had a good night's sleep. Actually, she feels exhausted all the time.

Social isolation

Patients with chronic pain typically withdraw from social activities. They are unable to continue working and leave their jobs. They eventually lose contact with friends, and family relations may become strained. They may have economic problems, having reduced income and increased spending on medication and special aids (mattress, crutches, pillows, cervical collars, etc.). They may also be funding more and more investigations and treatments, and are increasingly frustrated and despairing. The patient becomes typically cemented in a passive role 'Someone must be able to help me', and increasingly disillusioned with the health system and the social services.

Mrs Smith does not go out much any more. She's too tired, and the pain is always there. Her husband is quite irritable these days, he doesn't like her taking all the tablets and just lying in a chair in the evenings. He has to go on the evening walk alone. And he has to do the vacuuming, which he dislikes intensely. He has started going over to a friend's house, so that Mrs Smith is often alone in the evenings.

The patient has now become entangled in a very painful 'bad circle' where a host of factors are contributing to the pain and causing it to become overwhelming. The challenge for the therapist will be to determine the components of the individual pain experience, and especially which areas need to be addressed in order for the pain to be less painful.

Clinical and laboratory examination

Hans-Jacob Haga

History

Patterns of symptom expression will often be the key clues to the diagnosis. The physician must, therefore, both know the right questions and approach the patient in a patient-centered manner. Often, patients have made their own diagnoses and just want confirmation. This may be a challenge to the patient–doctor relationship. A careful, focused history that covers medical, social, and behavioral areas is important to elucidate important clues or patterns (Box 2.4).

Clinical examination

When patients present symptoms of muscular pain, it is important to make a proper clinical examination and evaluation in order to consider the various diagnostic possibilities. The duration of the complaints is of importance for

---

Box 2.4   *Summary of history*

- Hobbies, sports, profession, social clues, stress factors

- Initial symptoms

- Onset, localization, influence

- Evolution
  - *stationary*
  - *changing*: reference of pain, shifting, expanding
  - *recurrences*

- Patterns
  - *inflammatory*: nocturnal, morning stiffness
  - *mechanical*: starting pain, moving, during loading

- Other symptoms, including depression

- Functional disability

- Medication

- Coping strategies

- Family's attitudes to patient's pain

---

considering acute vs chronic conditions such as fibromyalgia, and so is the localization of the pain which in fibromyalgia is more generalized than in inflammatory rheumatic diseases and localized myalgia. A history with lack of effect on these symptoms by treatment with non-steroidal anti-inflammatory drugs, analgesics and physiotherapy is also of importance, indicating the presence of myofascial pain or fibromyalgia, since these therapeutic modalities usually have significant effect on inflammatory rheumatic diseases. Morning stiffness is common but not a specific sign of inflammatory rheumatic diseases, also being present in fibromyalgia and localized pain syndromes, but relief of pain and stiffness by moderate physical exercise is usually observed in inflammatory rheumatic diseases, with less impact in fibromyalgia. Muscular weakness may be secondary to pain, but is also a strong indication of muscular dysfunction which must be further examined for myositis, neuropathy and other myopathies. The presence of muscular atrophy or fibrillation strongly supports the diagnosis of a muscular or neurological disorder. The finding of sensory loss or pain in a localized dermatome or along the distribution of a well-defined nerve is also a strong indication of a neurological disorder. Pain in muscles experienced after firm pressure by the examiner or by exercise is often a non-specific finding and symptom, but is of importance for the diagnosis of fibromyalgia. In fibromyalgia, the presence of tender points is required for the diagnosis, in addition to a history of long-standing general muscular pain. Classification criteria for various rheumatic disorders like fibromyalgia are often designed for scientific purposes, however, and are therefore not always suitable as a diagnostic tool in clinical practice.

Differential diagnosis

Fibromyalgia and localized myalgia are common, but must be considered *after* other diagnostic possibilities, such as inflammatory rheumatic diseases, are ruled out (Box 2.5). Early diagnosis of inflammatory rheumatic diseases is of

---

Box 2.5 *Differential diagnoses to be considered in chronic myofascial pain (arthritis not demonstrated)*

- Fibromyalgia
- Localized myalgia
- Tenosynovitis/bursitis
- Neurological disorders
  - *nerve entrapment*
  - *cervical root affection*
- Thyroid disorders
- Hyperparathyroid disorders*
- Inflammatory rheumatic diseases
  - systemic lupus erythematosus*
  - Sjögren's syndrome
  - AS
  - myositis*
  - vasculitis*
  - polymyalgia rheumatica

* uncommon

---

great therapeutic and prognostic importance, and many of these diseases have a peak incidence between 30 and 50 years of age, which is also a peak incidence of myofascial pain.

The hallmark of most inflammatory rheumatic diseases is the finding of arthritis in one or several joints. The joints are tender and swollen with limited range of passive motion in all directions in a capsular pattern. In large joints, such as the hip and the shoulder, swelling is difficult to assess, and in these joints arthritis is suspected when there is a restricted range of passive motion in all directions associated with pain. A history of swollen joints reported by the patient should not be an indication of arthritis, as patients with fibromyalgia often report diffuse swelling of fingers and toes without clinical findings.

Patients with arthritis should be referred to a specialist in rheumatology without delay for early diagnosis. Patients without verified arthritis could still have an inflammatory rheumatic disease, as arthritis may be fluctuating in connective tissue diseases. More careful clinical and laboratory examination will therefore be necessary to exclude this possibility.

Patients with myofascial pain often complain about pain in the chest region. The same type of pain is often reported in patients with systemic lupus erythematosus (SLE) and primary Sjögren's syndrome (pSS) and is often caused by pleurisy. Pleurisy is rarely verified by clinical examination or x-ray investigation, and is usually fluctuating in contrast to the more or less constant pain experienced by patients with myofascial pain. Pleurisy is usually not associated with muscular pain. Almost all patients with SLE have various skin manifestations, and the most common manifestations at diagnosis are butterfly rash, photosensitivity and discoid lupus. Blood tests are often abnormal in SLE with anemia, high ESR and positive test for antinuclear antibodies (ANA). Practically all patients with pSS have symptoms of dry eyes or dry mouth, and they usually do not spontaneously inform their doctor about these problems as they are considered to be of less importance. The prevalence of pSS may be as high as 1% in the population, and most patients are women diagnosed at the age of 45 to 60 years. They usually see their doctor for unspecific symptoms such as myalgia, arthralgia and fatigue, and it is uncommon that they spontaneously complain about dryness of eyes and mouth. Patients with myalgia/arthralgia should therefore be interviewed about the sensation of dry eyes and/or mouth, and referred to an ophthalmologist if reporting about dry eyes. If there is no objective evidence of dry eyes, the diagnosis of pSS is unlikely. Our experience is that about half of the pSS patients have normal blood tests such as hemoglobin, ESR, and CRP - making these tests less suitable for screening for pSS. The finding of high ESR and normal CRP may indicate the presence of a connective tissue disease such as SLE or pSS, however, and further investigations should then be conducted by a rheumatologist.

Many patients with myofascial pain complain about chest pains, and therefore ankylosing spondylitis (AS) should also be considered. AS is usually diagnosed before the age of 40 years, and there is a male predominance. The dominant symptom of AS is low back pain at night and early in the morning improved by light exercise, in addition to chest pain with limited chest expansion. The diagnosis is verified by x-ray examination of the sacroiliac joints.

Thyroid disease should be considered in women with diffuse and widespread muscle pain. The muscle pains could precede clinically manifest thyroid disease by months and sometimes years, and they can persist for a long time after adequate treatment for the thyroid disease has been started. Hyperparathyroidism may also be associated with muscle pain, and therefore serum calcium and phosphate should be analysed. Another possibility to consider in CMP is neurological disease such as entrapment neuropathies and cervical root affection. A careful neurological examination should be considered, and in case of positive findings, further examinations by x-rays of columna should be done, eventually supplemented by CT or MR scans.

Patients with myofascial pain often complain about pain in both shoulders which could be due to local tenosynovitis or bursitis. Patients with CMP are predisposed to such conditions, and long-standing tenosynovitis predisposes to more widespread and chronic pain. Inflammation of the subacromial bursa or rotator cuff tendons may cause a 'painful arc' during abduction of the shoulder. The initial movement is painless, but from 90° the movement causes pain. When the arm reaches full abduction the pain ceases. Inflammation of the infraspinatus tendon is tested by resisted external rotation giving rise to pain. Inflammation of the subscapularis tendon is performed by resisted internal rotation of the shoulder, giving rise to more pain in the subacromial region. Inflammation of the supraspinatus tendon is performed by resisted abduction thereby increasing the pain felt in the subacromial region.

The most well-defined chronic myalgic pain syndrome is fibromyalgia. A consensus document on fibromyalgia in 1992 defined it as 'a painful, non-articular condition predominantly involving muscles'. It is also associated with exaggerated tenderness, fatigue, non-refreshing sleep and generalized stiffness in addition to several other bodily symptoms. According to the ACR 1990 criteria for the classification of fibromyalgia, there should be a history of widespread pain, and pain in 11 of 18 tender-point sites on digital palpation (Wolfe *et al.*, 1990). Widespread pain must have been present for at least three months, and the presence of a second clinical disorder does not exclude the diagnosis of fibromyalgia.

Laboratory examination

Serological screening for inflammatory rheumatic diseases is usually of limited value for family physicians, but may be of diagnostic importance for the rheumatologist. Most of the autoantibodies have low specificity, being specific in only a few disorders, such as the anti-DNA and anti-SM autoantibodies being diagnostic for SLE.

Other rare inflammatory rheumatic diseases such as vasculitis and myositis may be associated with diffuse muscular pain, and these patients are usually quite ill, with signs and symptoms indicating a serious disease. As outlined above, screening for thyroid disease and parathyroid disease should be performed, in addition to ordinary laboratory tests. It is of importance to note that ESR may be normal in inflammatory rheumatic diseases.

Fibromyalgia and myofascial pain are characterized by lack of abnormality in laboratory or radiological examinations. X-ray examination of the sacroiliac joints is mandatory in the diagnosic evaluation of AS.

Mrs Smith

The symptoms presented by Mrs Judith Smith suggest a diagnosis of localized chronic myofascial pain. Her long-standing problems do not exclude the possibility of an inflammatory rheumatic disorder, however, and further clinical examination and screening blood tests should be conducted as outlined above. Mrs Smith has no widespread pain above and below the waist and, therefore, she does not fulfill the criteria for fibromyalgia at this stage. She should be further examined for thyroid disease which often is associated with muscular pain.

References

Bongers PM, de Winter CR, Kompier MAJ and Hildebrandt VH (1993) Psychosocial factors at work and musculoskeletal disease. *Scand J Work Environ Health*. **19**: 297–312.

Bortz WM (1984) The disuse syndrome. *West J Med*. **141**: 691–9.

Brox JI, Røe C, Saugen E and Vøllestad NK (1997) Isometric abduction muscle activation in patients with rotator tendinosis of the shoulder. *Arch Phys Med Rehabil*. **78**: 1260–7.

Coderre TJ, Katz J, Vaccarino AL and Melzack R (1993) Contribution of central neuroplasticity to pathological pain: review of clinical and experimental evidence. *Pain*. **52**: 259–85.

Cook AJ, Woolf CJ, Wall PD and McMahon SB (1987) Expansion of cutaneous receptive fields of dorsal horn neurons following C-primary afferent fibre inputs. *Nature*. **325**: 151–3.

Crombez G, Eccleston C, Baeyens F and Eelen P (1998) When somatic information threatens, catastrophic thinking enhances attentional interference. *Pain*. **75**: 187–98.

Crombez G, Vlaeyen JW, Heuts P and Lysens R (1999) Pain-related fear is more disabling than pain itself: evidence on the role of pain-related fear in chronic back pain disability. *Pain*. **80**: 329–39.

Ejlertsen E, Andersen HB, Eliasen K and Mogensen T (1992) A comparison between preincisional and post-incisional lidocaine infiltration and post-operative pain. *Anesth Analg.* **74**: 495–8.

Fernandez E and Turk DC (1995) The scope and significance of anger in the experience of chronic pain. *Pain.* **612**: 165–75.

Fordyce WE (1976) *Behavioral Methods for Chronic Pain and Illness.* CV Mosby, St. Louis, MO.

Goldberg RT, Pachas WN and Keiths D (1999) Relationship between traumatic events in childhood and chronic pain. *Disabil Rehabil.* **21**: 23–30.

Hagberg M, Silverstein B, Wells R *et al.* (1995) *Work-related Musculoskeletal Disorders (WMSDs): a reference book for prevention.* Taylor & Francis, London, UK.

Kato J, Ogawa S, Katz J *et al.* (2000) Effects of pre-surgical local infiltration of bupivacaine in the surgical field on post-surgical wound pain in laparoscopic gynecologic examinations: a possible pre-emptive analgesic effect. *Clin J Pain.* **16**: 12–17.

Katz J, Kavanagh BP, Sandler AN *et al.* (1992) Pre-emptive analgesia: clinical evidence of neuroplasticity contributing to post-operative pain. *Anesthesiology.* **77**: 439–46.

Kjær M, Secher NH, Bach FW and Galbo H (1987) Role of motor center activity for hormonal changes and substrate mobilization in humans. *Am J Physiol.* **253**(22): R687–R695.

Le Bars D, Dickenson AH and Besson J-M (1979) Diffuse noxious inhibitory controls (DNIC) I: effects on dorsal horn convergent neurons in the rat. *Pain.* **6**: 283–304.

McCaul D and Malott JM (1984) Distraction and coping with pain. *Psychol. Bull.* **95**: 516–33.

Melzack R (1999) From the gate to the neuromatrix. *Pain Suppl.* **6**: S121–S126.

Melzack R and Wall PD (1965) Pain mechanisms: a new theory. *Science.* **150**: 971–9.

Russel IJ (1996) *Clinical Overview and Pathogenesis of the Fibromyalgia Syndrome, Myofascial Pain Syndrome, and Other Pain Syndromes.* Haworth Medical Press, New York.

Sejersted OM and Vøllestad NK (1993) Physiology of muscle fatigue and associated pain. In: H Værøy and H Merskey (eds) *Progress in Fibromyalgia and Myofascial Pain.* Elsevier Science Publishers, Amsterdam.

Svendsen F, Tjølsen A and Hole K (1998) AMPA and NMDA receptor-dependent spinal LTP after nociceptive tetanic stimulation. *Neuroreport.* **9**: 1185–90.

Turk DC (1996) Biopsychosocial perspective on chronic pain. In: RJ Gatchel and DC Turk (eds) *Psychological Approaches to Pain Management.* The Guilford Press, New York.

Ursin H, Endresen IM, Håland EM and Mjellem N (1993) Sensitization: a neurobiological theory for muscle pain. In: H Værøy and H Merskey (eds) *Progress in Fibromyalgia and Myofascial Pain.* Elsevier Science Publishers BV, Amsterdam.

Vøllestad NK, Sejersted I and Saugen E (1997) Mechanical behavior of skeletal muscle during intermittent voluntary isometric contractions in humans. *J Appl Physiol.* **83**: 1557–65.

Wall PD and Woolf CJ (1984) Muscle but not cutaneous C-afferent input produces prolonged increases in the excitability of the flexion reflex in the rat. *J Physiol (London).* **356**: 443–58.

Willis WD (1993) Mechanical allodynia: a role for sensitized nociceptive tract cells with convergent input from mechanoreceptors and nociceptors? *Am Pain Soc J.* **2**: 23–33.

Wolfe F, Smythe HA, Yunus MB *et al.* (1990) The American College of Rheumatology 1990 criteria for the classification of fibromyalgia. *Arthritis Rheum.* **33**: 160–72.

3

The illness experience

The pain is an everlasting reminder for Judith Smith that her body feels worn out. The pain is all over her body, never giving her an hour of rest. Sometimes, it seeps into every muscular fiber, threatening her with the thought that something serious must be wrong. Judith had a close friend with rheumatoid arthritis who died last year from breast cancer. You never know what might be wrong when it hurts so badly.

Judith is a little overweight and not very proud of her appearance, and she really feels old. She is well aware of how the pain can be related to her workload at the laundry and at home, but is not in charge of changing the conditions that produce the stress. When she comes home from work, there is still a lot to be done in the house. In spite of the pain and her tiredness, she strives to keep her home neat and tidy. It is especially hard work because the floors need to be repaired.

Greg was never used to doing women's work, and he is so busy. Judith takes care of him and the children. She blames herself for always being so obliging, always taking responsibility for everything and everybody, as all the small chores together wear her out, but at the same time, she is proud to contribute. 'How could a hospital exist without a laundry?' she asks smiling, 'And how would Greg survive without my cooking?'.

The first component of the patient-centered clinical method requires the physician to explore both the disease and the illness experience. The history, physical examination and lab tests are usually accomplished by the physician without major hesitation. However, further attention is needed to make sure that patients' ideas, feelings, expectations and ability are incorporated and given priority. In clinical work, illness experience may differ from, or even contradict, the physician's biomedical assumptions and images that shape his or her agenda and approach. Encounters with patients suffering from CMP and other medically unexplained conditions challenge the physician's understanding of bodily phenomena and demonstrate shortcomings of a strictly biomedical base of knowledge. In such cases, a thorough understanding of the patient's agenda is essential for the physician to set the stage for finding common ground. In this chapter, we shall learn more about the meaning and impact of the illness experience in patients with chronic pain, and suggest some pathways for getting access to patient narratives.

Communicating illness experience

Per Stensland

An illness narrative takes time to develop and may need a favorable situation to emerge. Setting the scene for a favorable situation is a task for the health-care provider. The physician's most powerful 'drug' when setting this scene is himself/herself and his/her relation to the patient (Balint, 1964). One of the challenges for the physician may be described as making space in the consultation for the patient's subjective experience and contextual information from his/her everyday life. This calls for a patient-centered expansion of the focus of the medical dialogue (Stewart *et al.*, 1995). Below, I will share some experiences and reflections from clinical practice and action research. The research approach is further presented in Chapter 6.

Towards a personal description of pain

When patients are given the opportunity to present their stories thoroughly in their own words, the illness narrative may sound fresh to the listener. This may give new clues to clinically relevant information concerning the symptom itself, accompanying complaints and the situations where they appear.

> A young man of 23 attended his physician because of pain in his chest. He had had his pain medically evaluated two years ago, but now it was worse. He said, 'My life is falling apart, I am always tired, I can't think and I hardly eat.' He told his physician that for the last six months, he had also developed sleep disturbances and dizziness. He was in danger of losing his factory job due to absence. And what he ate was nothing but junk food. The pain was a part, but only a part, of the problem. Helping him presupposed an approach that embraced his medical problem, work problem, eating habits and maybe more. The family physician would get a chance to reassess the effect of the first interventions when the patient returned.

Another man, 54 years old, with a physically strenuous job, had for many years been complaining of pain in his chest, neck and shoulders. He had been seen at the hospital several times, going through x-ray examinations and cardiac check-ups. He said, 'As all these results are okay, I guess you think I'm okay, but I'm not. These pains bother me a lot, like an ever-present, open wound. So I have no choice but to be worried.' The patient's lively description made me as his primary care physician curious enough to continue investigations and find a hitherto misinterpreted cardiac disease.

A patient-centered approach may provide information to sharpen the diagnosis, simply by turning general descriptions into more personal terms. Dialogues that expand the information base may alter the problem formulation. Medical complaints may turn out to be less frequent, less significant, or quite different when they have been subject to patient-centered co-operation in the consultation. Many patients report that an invitation to share personal information has strengthened their relation to the physician.

Gaining access to the insight of the patient

The patient's own insight into her illness experience can be expressed as an illness story. However, the story told by the patient may compete with alternative narratives about the same condition, such as is illustrated by a woman of 24, who experienced her only back-ache attack during the preceding month during an eight-hour drive with her mother. When she initially presented her complaint, she remembered only the quality of her back ache. Being given the opportunity to take a step back and reflect on her symptoms, she shared an experience that placed her complaints in another context, where her relationship with her mother was a key point. Her symptom now had a new meaning, and the physician obtained access to connections between her illness and her life.

Joe, a 12-year-old boy, had been treated in the hospital for a headache that had bothered him seriously for a year. His attacks were dramatic; they seemed difficult to predict and they interfered with school and physical activity. They were understood and treated as a migraine, though the effect of treatment was not convincing. In a consultation where his mother (M) participated, this conversation between Joe (J) and the physician (P) took place:
P: *What happened?*
J: *It was the first time I felt something before it started.*
P: *And what did you feel?*

J: *I felt like a sting in my neck!*
P: *It started like a sting . . .*
J: *Mm*
P: *And do you remember anything that may have started this attack?*
J: *No . . . it just came*
P: *It just came . . .*
M: *I thought you might be anxious about our holiday*
J: *No, I wasn't*
M: *I thought so*
P: *So you don't think that it is possible to imagine that this had got anything to do with anxiety.*
J: *No*
P: *It had not*
J: *I was not anxious . . . I was sad . . . because I didn't get any new clothes for the holiday like my brothers did.*

A consultation based on Joe's own understanding of his complaint focused on context and family rather than medication. Joe himself concluded: 'I don't know what kind of disease this is, if it is a disease. Maybe it is some kind of stress.'

Patients have personal expressions to describe their complaints or symptoms. The color of these descriptions and metaphors gives additional information on how the patient sees his or her situation. If you are 'stiff as a stick', this may give you lumbar pain, but may also prevent you from being flexible.

Exploring internal dialogues and locked voices

By the time a sense of illness is formulated to others, it has already developed in a private or internal conversation. Worries, fears or ideas of mastering a problem come to the mind of the patient as voices of different quality (Vygotsky, 1988).

Peter, a 36-year-old man was injured in an accident in which another person was also badly hurt. He got a whiplash neck strain with ensuing headache, neck pain and sleep disturbances. Two years later he was still on partial sick leave.
Physician: *When waking up with pain, you may sometimes find an idea flying through your mind or hear yourself saying something. When you wake up at night, what kind of ideas come to you?*
Peter: *Well . . . no . . . I get angry . . . 'cause my whole life is actually a failure . . . and what I get mad about . . . is that I don't seem to get well, and I feel totally innocent . . . and I don't feel certain about what is bothering me . . .*

The personal meaning of waking up with pain became clearer for this patient as well as the physician. Aspects of guilt were otherwise firmly rejected by this troubled man, but they were apparent in the ensuing conversation. The internal dialogues added aspects of time and authenticity, bringing the 'moment of pain' to the consultation.

Anna was a 27-year-old student teacher when she suffered a head injury, giving her a minor concussion. After four years she was still seriously bothered by head and neck pain both at work and in her private life:

A: *I just feel like an outsider . . . I have lost the pleasure in my life. This headache is grumbling all the time . . .*

P: *When experiencing or waking up with this pain, what kind of ideas are flying through your mind? What do you say to yourself?*

A: *Cheer up, cheer up! Nothing is wrong with you! But something is wrong with me! I simply believe that people can notice it . . . that this pain can be seen outside. At any rate, something has changed completely. I used to stand up, be elected for this and that. I wanted it like that. Now I don't want anything, don't dare anything . . .*

Anna was trying to combat her feeling of having lost her pleasure. The struggling is giving her a feeling of being alien, which may contribute to her already difficult situation. Her internal dialogues display the quality, the color and life of her fight against giving up.

Presenting one's story to the physician

Forming and informing

Sharing the illness narrative means meeting the other face to face. As each individual is unique, the frame of each meeting is novel. The encounter gives an opportunity to formulate, express and hear how one's message sounds. When a boy of 12 with a feeble voice tells the physician and his mother that he does not feel he is properly 'seen' by his parents, the boy may see how his words fall by watching our faces, showing him what kind of statement this is. (Are we touched? Did he manage to express himself so that we heard what he hoped we should hear?)

The specific meaning of his words in spoken language is shown through and by the articulation of his message. His respiration, intonation and gesture constitute a language that conveys a surplus of information, the surplus that shows what he means when he means more than he says. The articulation of some words may be seen to touch him, as a story is informing the speaker as much as it is informing the listener (Andersen, 1995). The physician hears both through ear and eye 'listening', and is actively participating in shaping the self-image of the speaker; encouraging or discouraging what may be said.

The 'internal voice' metaphor

Human thinking may metaphorically be seen as a dialogue between internal voices (Vygotsky, 1988). Recollecting a conversation, like hearing oneself saying what 'should have been said', may remind us of how we go about having dialogues, preparing for or handling the effect of events encountered in life. The experience of body symptoms may give rise to 'self-talk'. The appearance of internal dialogues may be brief and sometimes inaccessible if they are not actively requested, as with the person who felt 'innocent' about his accident. This connection to the moment of pain gives the internal voices a way to open access to authentic storytelling. Attending to and modifying these voices is a process of dialogue, which may be utilized in medicine.

When illness has been present for a long time, the internal dialogues may have changed to monotonous and negative monologues (Penn and Frankfurt, 1994), as the voice that told the worried man that his life was a failure. By giving access to alternative internal voices, a dialogue on long-standing symptoms may contribute to move repetitive internal, negative monologues from a fixed position to a less fixed one, to internal, positive dialogues.

> When Judith Smith (JS) consults her physician (P) he asks her to keep an illness diary. She returns after four weeks.
>
> **P:** *Okay, it's a month since you were here and, let's see (reads) ... you have made a note about chest pain nearly every day ... It seems to have been bad here ...*
>
> **JS:** *It's quite strange to write it down like that ...*
>
> **P:** *You have taken less tablets than you used to ... 10 tablets in a month, that is less than half of what you previously took. Two pills a week.*
>
> **JS:** *Uh, I have tried not to take anything, but at times I need something. This diary makes me kind of more aware than before. Still ... that does not mean that I'm okay.*
>
> **P:** *Hm, you have made a note on how this feels; you feel it in every muscle in your chest ...*
>
> **JS:** *Sure, I never get rest, it's creeping around in my body.*
>
> Judith described a voice that accompanied her chest pain. The physician asked her later to make notes on what the voice tells her.

P: *Here you start writing about two kinds of voices.*

JS: *Yes, you see, I also have another voice, a small black one, and maybe that voice is more prominent than the good, white one. Yes, I think so . . . the black one is there all the time, tells me about uneasiness and says: You won't manage . . . I think he . . . no, I mean (laughs) it . . . is much easier to find than the good one . . .*

Hearing a white voice inside may feel different from hearing a black one. The negative, repetitive character of this voice that accompanied her symptom might represent an additional tension, or perhaps the very burden of her headache. The voice had a gender, indicating that it echoed or resembled the voice of a specific person whom the patient knew. Judith later summed up her experience with making notes:

JS: *At times it was not easy to understand what I said . . . I don't think I wanted you to hear so much . . .*

P: *. . . At times one may prefer to keep words for oneself?*

JS: *I think you heard what I said, but you seemed to search for more information than I was ready to give.*

P: *And that was . . .*

JS: *I don't think I was ready to admit to myself how the quarrels with my daughter stole my energy.*

P: *But this became clearer to you?*

JS: *You know, we shed some light on this matter by talking, but I thought I would need more time, because I did not manage to talk so much about it, but then I had this paper, so I could write something down. And it was a bit easier then, when I came back and said 'here is the paper'. It talked somewhat more than I did . . .*

In her autobiographical novel, telling the story of how pain and disability changed her life, the poet Suzanne E Berger describes the profound consequences of being vulnerable, suffering and having to change all her essential preconditions for living a dignified life with chronic disease (Berger, 1996). In the mundane act of bending down, Suzanne Berger suffered a back injury so severe that she was left suddenly and dramatically disabled:

'The house of the body in pain is furnished with inexact metaphors that resist tidy medical labeling, and with approximate descriptions of extreme states. You find yourself at a loss, with language running dry just when needed most, that is, when explaining an internal, teeming microcosm to the medical world, the physical therapy world, and to the macrocosmic world of relationship to others in general. Since pain can neither be verified nor denied in many cases, the person in pain is doubted – are you malingering or over-dramatizing? – which only then amplifies the pain. With only vivid, but subjective comparisons to 'defend' ourselves with, we can hardly communicate at all. I remember saying, "It feels like my back is a radio someone took apart and put back the wrong way" to the wondering disbelief of the doctor attending to me.'

Women in pain: the meaning of symptoms and illness

Eva E Johansson and Katarina Hamberg

Women with chronic pain are often described as frustrating, vague and incomprehensible. To explore the reasons for these difficulties, we did a qualitative study based on repeated interviews with 20 Swedish women with CMP (Johansson, 1998; Johansson *et al.*, 1999). The aim was to extract what kind of information the women gave in the web of vague and rambling symptom descriptions.

An analysis of symptom descriptions

Analyzing what the women actually told about their pain, we realized that symptom descriptions are often tightly woven webs of different threads of information. Some threads are apparent and form clearly visible patterns. Others are only hinted at, and still others are hidden, although they may be very important for the structure and context. In the analysis of the interview data, numerous 'threads' were sorted out and grouped together as:

- feelings embedded in bodily presentations
- explanatory ideas
- consequences of pain in daily life
- consequences for identity and self.

A summary of the findings will be presented below and then discussed from a gender perspective.

But first of all, let us listen to the symptom description of Alice, a 40-year-old woman working as a cleaner.

'Well, this time it began in the fingers. I was sick, incredibly sick. And then I got this cramp. I lay down for 10 or 15 minutes at work that night, which

I never do. But I had terrible pains in the lungs. Fingers, too. I remember that when I was going to shift gears when I drove home I couldn't get my fingers around the stick and had to push the gear like this. Then it moved to the neck, and here behind the shoulder blade. A lump was stuck there and hurt. Then it moved. Since then it has gone up and down, actually. The slightest bit of exertion and it hurts again. And lately I think it has become worse. Today I feel really good. I just have a little pain in the neck. But I have it in my ankles, I have it in my hips, I have it in my thighs. I have it everywhere! But the cramp is actually a little better now. Otherwise it is everywhere. Which is why I thought that I might have got that disease, fibro...? Because it moves around so much. From one place to another. And the pain is so intense. Like last weekend, in the back of the neck and the fingers, so incredible, incredible ... then it goes up into the flesh itself, or however I should put it, and then in the back of the neck.'

Feelings embedded in the bodily presentations

The extensive symptom descriptions might initially appear as incomprehensible from a biomedical standpoint. For instance, just like Alice, many women described their bodies as detached into separate parts, not as a compound entity. 'My fingers are not obeying orders' or 'Suddenly my legs turned all crazy, I didn't recognize them as mine'. The bodily symptoms were therefore difficult to grasp and unpredictable for the woman herself. Some of the women felt like victims, as if 'it' (the pain) was a constantly present, but yet invisible enemy. 'Then it moved, and now it is located in . . .'. 'It' was an intruder, an alien visitor, out of her control, reminding her whenever she felt a little better. 'But the cramp is actually a little better now. Otherwise it's everywhere.'

Throughout the pain descriptions, most of the women questioned and worried about what the symptoms might be announcing. Pain was a serious threat of 'something going wrong' in the body, and they had to be on the watch for changes for the worse.

'Most of the nights I got up and wandered around the house at night and felt pain and it tingled and hurt ... I really thought I had some sort of serious neurological disease. I thought I had better pay close attention before I became paralyzed and lost my sense of touch, so that I could commit suicide before I turned into a vegetable.'

The bodily presentations, with the pain being everywhere and nowhere, better and worse, moving around, up and down, suggested feelings of deep worries and lack of control.

Explanatory ideas

All the women we spoke to were convinced that their pain had a physical origin. Medical diagnoses were often hinted at 'Could it be fibro . . .?', and further investigations were suggested, as if it was up to them to push and make claims if anything at all was to be done.

> 'There must be something concrete there, as I can feel it so strongly.'

An explanation near at hand for many of the women in the study, as for Judith Smith, was that they were worn-out. They thought the pain was caused by the heavy and monotonous situation at work, and was a result of repetitive strain injuries. 'I think it is job-related. I'm pretty sure of that.' Furthermore, the women had ideas about other environmental influences causing bodily damages. These explanations were the kind that are controversial within the biomedical framework, such as unfavorable influences of minerals or metals, such as amalgam or gold, of magnetism and radiation, and of the weather. However, when listening further about what the women told, the reported overstraining also seemed to appear as the consequence of household responsibilities and chores:

> 'I've done everything, I have, really! And managed all right. I have been janitor, mechanic, gardener and painter. So it's really not so strange that I should have pains in all my joints. One has to be so darned competent all the time.'

Many informants described how tensions and worries had elicited the strain that contributed to muscular pain. Stressful life events or living conditions were described, such as a stressful childhood, disagreements at the workplace and marital conflicts:

> 'Really, it's not strange that I'm tense and have pain. I always had to tiptoe, was always afraid and I never knew if I did the right thing and if he was content. When he began to harass our youngest son too, I moved.'

Images of pain as the punishment for wrong decisions, or even bad behavior were frequently presented. The pain was connected to feelings of being inadequate in relationships with parents-in-law, parents, husbands or children, not doing things she was expected to do. The women talked about guilt, but also grief and shame. This might involve a period of addiction to alcohol or tranquilizers, having been sexually abused or beaten, or having had an abortion:

> 'I kind of believe in fate. In a way you want to think that everything has a meaning. And I have had these thoughts that I was punished for having this abortion. That it was God's punishment that forced me to stop knitting, and weaving, and that my world collapsed.'

To summarize, the women thought they had a physical damage, a disease, elicited by long-time overstraining and stressful social circumstances. These ideas are not new or controversial. The problem for the women was that they felt that the disease was not recognized by the physicians, and that nobody seemed to be interested, or to be able to help.

Consequences of pain in daily life

Interwoven in the symptom descriptions were also examples of how the pain had consequences for everyday activities, at work, at home and during leisure time. The women evaluated their resources in relation to former capabilities and present expectations. Anita said:

'Well, you know. I wonder if I can ever go back to the job I had. I don't think so. The problems with my fingers, which you're so dependent on. I'll give you an example. Yesterday, the sun shone directly into my kitchen so that you saw everything clearly, the doors and everything. So automatically I got a rag and started cleaning. But as soon as I did, my fingers started hurting. Completely exhausted. Just that little thing. So one starts to think, how would I be able to manage a job, when I can't even do this? And I have to divide the apartment up into rooms when I vacuum. How then is one supposed to manage the heavy workload we have?'

In the example above, Anita described a housework routine that she evidently executed automatically and regarded as trivial. The domestic undertakings were core examples in many ways. They illustrated that sickness certification did not liberate women from housework. Expressed as reflexes, 'automatically I got a rag', these cleaning examples gave glimpses of this woman's life-world; what is expected from her, and what she expects from herself, i.e. what is socialized so deeply that it works on the spinal level. In their narratives the women formulated many of these taken-for-granted expectations:

'I have my better periods, you know. That's when I try to do everything that needs to be done. Like what? Well, I sew new curtains, I want to clean, and wipe out all the cupboards, in depth, and the things inside the cupboards, and . . . things I actually can't do now, you know? And so, as a result, afterwards I feel ten times worse.'

By the time the women were interviewed they were sick-listed, full-time or partly. Therefore, it was not strange that their descriptions of restricted work capacities were taken from the domestic arena. However, in general, when the women described their daily work they did not distinguish between unpaid and paid work. These women had jobs such as cleaners, nursing assistants, kitchen maids and child-minders. In fact, their paid work was often very similar to their duties at home. How the women acted when working life ambitions clashed with family concerns is further evolved in Chapter 4. Their ideas about how to prioritize had roots in experiences of social conventions. Birgitta was 61 years old and had worked as nursing assistant all her life:

> 'I've always said: If you give life to children it is your responsibility to take good care of them, too. When my children were little, I knew I didn't want to give up my job either. So, I worked nights, part-time, and looked after my children in the daytime. I know we discussed this, but my husband said it was impossible for him to cut down work hours for childcare. It was impossible to ask for at the building firm where he worked, he said.'

The pain had consequences for the women's caring duties; as daughters, mothers, wives or even grandmothers. For instance, one woman really felt ashamed of not being able to help her parents mend their towels and linen, as she was expected to do. A mother of two school-age children blamed herself for not having enough strength for playing and being nice. Another described how the insistent pain made her irritable. She feared being seen as only complaining and nagging by her husband and daughter, when she asked them to take part in the household chores. One of the grandmothers, in fact Birgitta, recounted how she had trouble finding acceptance for not involving herself with her grandchildren.

> 'The pain makes it hard to handle small children. My son and daughter-in-law ought to, but they don't accept it, in a way ... my illness. I feel stung; because I know there are people saying that grandchildren are the most wonderful experience on earth. I don't have that feeling. Is that horrible? I don't live up to the ideal grandma.'

The pain was described as an obstacle to performing paid work, domestic chores, and also activities that formerly had given pleasure, relaxation, and identity, for instance knitting, embroidering, berry-picking, weaving or running. Thereby the pain also had consequences for self-perception and self-esteem.

Consequences for identity and self

The pain, and its consequences, were perceived as a menace to the woman's reputation, risking her good name. To be suffering from something that did not show and could be medically diagnosed was a delicate issue to handle. A recurring theme was the uncertainty of how to interpret and deal with lowered working capacities in private life, at the workplace, and officially in terms of insurance rights. The women wanted 'to do', to be active and respected. However, in most circumstances they found themselves exposed to doubt and mistrust in the eyes of others.

This was a dilemma. Being at home and sick-listed, they felt expectations from others to take on 'extra responsibilities' and have a perfect home. At the same time, if they were active, went out shopping, cleaned windows, it could make the neighbors suspicious: If she was that able-bodied, why couldn't she manage to go to work?

> Betty, a 38-year-old barmaid, had been sick-listed for a year for widespread pain. Many work-trials had failed, and she considered herself incapable of taking part in the labor market. As far as the pain went, she was reconciled to living with it the rest of her life. She began planning to adopt a child. The adoption bureau needed a doctor's health certificate. She was utterly astonished, and insulted, when the agency hesitated to recommend adoption because of her decreased working capabilities. She tried to object on the grounds of the illness disqualifying her as a woman:

>> 'Although I'm sick-listed full-time for pain disorders, I'm a totally healthy woman and I would be a perfect mother.'

A few informants gave spontaneous information about the problems that the pain caused in their sex life. In doing this, they chose to describe their inadequacies towards their partner rather than their own expectations. Alice described her wish 'to do' as a wife, to be accessible for her husband's needs:

> 'And these pains affect sex life, too. It consumes a whole lot of the desire. And men are, well, like, they don't function the same way. If they have pain they still can function sexually. But I don't, so it can be a problem. But I see what it does to him, it puts him in a bad mood.'

What Betty and Alice exemplified went for the other women as well. When describing their disability and shortcomings in a way that made them understandable and legitimate, they risked being labeled, not only as malingerers, hypochondriacs or psychological deviants, but also as being insufficiently womanly. Their identities were being questioned.

Illness experiences read through a gender lens

Pain is a private experience to which no one else has direct access. When trying to understand patient experiences, we are dependent on what the sufferer tells us and how it is told. The tools to gain insight are to watch, listen and interpret what we see and hear, and to integrate it into our understanding. Doctors and patients have different agendas and therefore different ways of interpreting experiences. The patient-centered clinical method encourages the physician to try to enter the patient's world, and see the illness through the patient's eyes. Understanding the patient's expectations, feelings, and fears cannot be reached without allowing the patient to express all her reasons for attendance.

A gender perspective is neither the patient's nor the doctor's perspective, but an analytical viewpoint acknowledging that women and men have different experiences and strategies because of their biological, social, cultural, ethnic and political circumstances. A genderized analysis considers the 'gender order', i.e. in all human societies there is an over-ruling pattern where women are subordinate to men. The gender order is overtly displayed in statistics on income, position and power, and also exists in more hidden and variable forms. For each individual, man and woman alike, the personal experience exposes how the gender order is maintained, challenged, varied or changed. Much research has been done so far on gender and communication in medical consultations (*see* Chapter 5), but pain research still frequently lacks a gender analysis.

Myofascial pain disorders are frequent in the whole population, but women constitute the vast majority in most epidemiological studies, often two-thirds of the population suffering from chronic pain syndromes (*see* Chapter 1). There is no consistent physiological explanation for this, rather divergent theories on overuse, underuse or incorrect use of the locomotor system are discussed. There are also hypotheses that musculoskeletal complaints are the result of learned behavior or social inheritance. Gijsberg and Kolk (1997) discuss the fact that women in general utilize healthcare and report symptoms more extensively than men, as a result of early socialization, traditional sex roles and differences in social position. Bendelow (1993) contributed to the understanding of pain, gender, culture and embodiment in a study on pain endurance, by suggesting that lay health beliefs attributed superior capacity for endurance of pain in women as compared to men. Instead of acknowledging women's pain experiences and taking them seriously as such, suffering may be attributed to women's 'nature'.

One of the aims of our study was to understand the meaning of the pain experiences as interpreted by the patients themselves. The way the pain in the body was described, as a frightening threat, expressed powerlessness. They felt they lacked control over what happened in their own bodies, and expressed this as being victims of an unidentified disease. Yes, the patients expected that there was a disease, a physical damage behind the signaling pain. It was explained by long-time overstraining and stressful social circumstances, such as heavy workload, but also violence and abuse. The causal agents, too, were now out of their power to change. The perception of persistent damage was also there. The women were worn out for reasons for which no one could actually be held personally responsible. Still, since neither the causative factors nor the damage were recognized by the physicians, the women also blamed themselves. Furthermore, they also said that nobody seemed to be able to help, or was interested in trying. The pain itself, the lack of control and the resulting deadlock induced problems in everyday life that jeopardized the women's sense of self and their identities as capable women. They were not able to take full part in the labor force, nor to live up to expectations of themselves as daughters, wives and mothers.

Below, we will compare findings on the meaning of pain from our study with other research findings. In addition, we shall interpret these experiences from a perspective of power, subordination and gendered demands. We consider the women's symptom descriptions, their explanations and their consequences as dependent on the social context of the women, such as family members, friends, neighbors, co-workers and healthcare providers.

Lack of control

'Control' is not a new concept in pain theories, but appears frequently in cognitive therapeutic models. Banyard and Graham-Bermann (1993) remark that prevailing theories about coping are usually formulated on the basis of the individual's cognition, his or her personality and functioning, as if such characteristics were untouched by gender, race and class. Value judgments used for interpretation of coping strategies (what is considered as 'good' or 'bad' coping) are problematic for any studies of women's lives. Women always fall on the lower end of the coping hierarchy. For instance, it is thought that people with high 'self-efficacy beliefs' have fewer shortcomings in their life, while people who react with 'helplessness' and 'relying on others' enhance their suffering and medical help-seeking (Jensen *et al.*, 1991). With this perspective, poor outcome in terms of rehabilitation is explained by the individual's 'catastrophizing' mode, 'pain behavior' (Jensen *et al.*, 1994), or even pain-prone personality.

According to such explanation models, women's failures in rehabilitation as compared to men should then depend on differences of personalities. There is, however, a risk here of confounding origin and outcome. For instance, we might imagine that an unsuccessful rehabilitation period could foster a pain-prone behavior. So far, we conclude that there are no simple cause–effect relations, but complex patterns of inter-related factors involved in the sources and consequences of pain when it comes to gender and rehabilitation. It is also possible that different circumstances for women and men in rehabilitation programs can explain the differences in outcome. Traditional coping theories pay no attention to the fact that women employ different strategies from men, such as negotiation, indulgence, empathy or social support.

Although the women in our study told stories about lack of control, we did not interpret it as a personality state or a depression. From a gender perspective, a more plausible explanation was that this could be due to low access to resources and power. Our informants were mostly working-class or lower middle-class women, who were subordinated at work and in healthcare. Although they reported high levels of bodily awareness, they did not have the chance to apply this insight through modification of their working life and private life. Gijsberg and Kolk (1997) have suggested that women's greater tendency to attribute bodily sensations to somatic illness can be due to gender-specific socialization.

Victims of an unexplained disease

The women came up with many different explanations of their myofascial pain. Nevertheless, the majority ended up fearing disease and physiological damage:

'I don't think it is merely psychological, as I feel it in my body, and that frightens me.'

We consider health and illness as socially constructed notions, that mean different things to different people. In CMP, there may be discrepancies between diseases and illness behavior and lack of consensus among lay people and healthcare professionals. Research has demonstrated how, while patients try to verify the reality of the pain and its physical origin, they search for the still-undiscovered disease. Confirmation of a diagnosis such as fibromyalgia may bring relief (Raymond & Brown, 2000). Physicians, on the other hand, tend to consider chronic pain as a dysfunctional reaction (Eccleston *et al.*, 1997).

This commonly occurring discrepancy represents an important challenge for the patient-centered approach, underlining the significance of obtaining access to the illness experience of the patient. Throughout the Western world, biophysical facts are given primacy over human interpretations. We believe this is one of the major sources of misunderstanding and distrust between patient and physician. The biomedical dualism between body and soul permeates not only lay beliefs, but also beliefs in medicine, politics and welfare legislation. The popular press provides cultural imprints on the cultural images of women's symptoms, by bringing advice to women on such health complaints as premenstrual syndrome, fibromyalgia or CFS.

Social insurance rules are also mediating the dismissal of subjective symptoms where objective findings cannot be identified by the physician. In Sweden, a medical diagnosis must be obtained before a sick certificate can be granted. The close relationship between medicine and welfare benefits through diagnosis explains why a diagnosis is utterly important for the patient to perceive themselves as justified and taken seriously. In our study, the women spelled out how essential it was to get a credible explanation for their pain: 'I was willing to be cut in pieces to figure out what was wrong with me.' The women worked hard to maintain their self-respect by acquiring a name for the disorder, in order to be able to collaborate against it. We suggest that more time and concentration from the physician must be invested in acknowledging this issue, by incorporating the patient's own explanations into the medical understanding of the illness manifestations.

However, focusing merely on diagnosis, just to provide an acceptable label, might also become a deadlock. High levels of investigation and treatment of chronic pain, including surgery, that are carried out along the technical and interventional track of Western medicine can only provide short-time reassurance for patient and physician. The research findings we have presented so far emphasize the need to extend the traditional explanatory models of medicine. The physician's awareness may be enhanced by realizing how illness perceptions and behavior in men and women are shaped in cultural and social moulds. Pain is a lived experience in daily-life undertakings. To legitimize this experience, to give the right information, and reinforce the self-appraisal of the patient, the everyday life conditions must be made visible. As Mechanic states: 'Sickness in a social sense could be a vehicle of power and influence, making new adaptations possible' (Mechanic, 1995).

Jeopardizing womanliness through a life in pain

We have already heard about the consequences of pain in determining self-identity for this group of women patients. Certain verbal expressions heard in our study, such as 'one should and would', illustrated not only general moralities and social norms, but also representations of gendered guides to what the women considered to be expected from a capable woman, i.e. a 'real' woman.

Disabilities in household chores and problems in fulfilling family commitments were frequently mentioned by the women in our study. It was striking and surprising for us, as women and researchers and physicians, that so many of the women (independent of age) used vacuum cleaning as an example to talk about their physical capacity. From clinical practice, we notice that men usually talk about lawn mowing or snow shoveling when they describe their capacity and shortcomings. We can observe how the metaphors related to illness experience are contextual and gender-related. The consequences of pain on identity appear to be closely connected to gender roles or even stereotypes, and these in turn are related to social class.

The women in our study told about their perceived social expectations of womanliness as related to cleaning, caring and accessibility for others' needs.

This seemed to multiply and perhaps create ambiguities for the consequences of illness: in order to be respected as women, they had to fulfill the norms of household work. However, by doing so, they risked being mistrusted. These findings confirm essential concepts identified by Borkan and co-workers, such as limitations and delegitimization in the lives of patients (Borkan *et al.*, 1995). Although drawn from a study on women patients, we suggest that these principles may be transferable to men. In order to keep an intact 'manliness', a man will have to maintain sport interest, hunting, fishing, car mending and independence. However when doing so, his neighbors mistrust his illness, and also himself.

In our study, stories about tensions and worries or shame and guilt were not only read as examples of self-blame, but also as features of being in a vulnerable situation. This impression was supported when the women themselves seemed to conceal or verbally reformulate their subordination. For instance, during the first interviews, only two of the women unveiled experiences of abuse. However, by the time of the third interview, as many as half of the women had spoken about experiences of physical abuse (*see* Chapter 4).

Each individual woman described internal voices and inner dialogues that compared and considered former and present abilities and her emotional state, in relation to normative conditions: How shall I expend my resources and adapt to my limitations? What can I do at home? Am I capable of working, or entitled to be sick-listed? How am I considered in the eyes of family members, neighbors and doctors? What was taken for normal and natural, and what was considered as illness?

In addition to their tasks as medical advisers, physicians are very important legitimizing agents. When it concerns patients with chronic pain, we think there is a need to ask whether physicians are aware and prepared for such an assignment. A purely diagnosis-oriented approach is not enough. Using the patient-centered clinical method, an attitude of healing through adaptation must be adopted with a gender perspective on women's and men's actual circumstances, expectations and values. From an understanding of these matters, physicians may have a chance to see, listen, voice concern, discuss solutions and offer remedies, as well as medication, to empower the patient.

Our study disclosed clues in the women's narratives where follow-up questions could open up to inner, hidden feelings, fears and expectations. For instance, conditional conjunctions such as 'if only ... I would' and the use of the indefinite pronoun 'one' demonstrated the gaps between the actual circumstances and societal ideals, between personal capacities and what they felt was expected of them. By referring to the standards of housewives and mothers, the women themselves assigned their main arena, and its delimitation. The subtle utterance 'The sun shone directly into my kitchen . . .' signaled a world of having an eye for essential duties, that might be invisible for some but mandatory for the actual woman. This woman articulates her goals and attempts, inhibited by bodily pain: 'What I'd really like to do . . . sew curtains, clean out the cupboards.'

Although the origin of pain might be physical and psychosocial, its persistence can be traced through life conditions, norms and gender-related tasks, which often remain disguised during the consultation. The consultation is only a small part of the patient's total life situation. Still, exploring the patient perspective, while also considering the impact of gender in everyday life and in the consultation context, could be the start of the healing process.

Judith Smith is scared by her pain, and feels that she has lost control over what happens in her body. She feels as if she is being invaded by an alien intruder, who hits her whenever she feels a little better. It sucks the spirit out of her, and she wonders what's the matter with her. What has she done to deserve this unease? Late at night, dark thoughts turn up and she blames herself for that abortion, although it was long ago. Tensions and worries might, perhaps, get stuck in muscle fibers?

The continuous limitations caused by the pain make her feel so belittled. She used to consider herself a busy bee, capable of everything, managing work and still having strength left for laughs and hospitality at home. Now she can't keep up the standards she wants to have at home and hates the thought of the critical eyes of visitors. Formerly easy things, like keeping the house neat and tidy, are now heavy duties. Saturday her sister-in-law is coming to visit, and she will look around. The dust is growing, and vacuum cleaning is certainly not something she can ask Greg or the children to do. He is busy with fixing the boat for a weekend picnic, and the kids have their school work to do. She feels no understanding from her relatives, just expectations. 'You ought to pull yourself together; who hasn't got pain?' is a standard answer when she tries to explain. Then it is hard to confide in them, so she tries to keep up the façade and manage in front of everyone, even the doctor. If he only could imagine her situation!

References

Andersen T (1995) Reflecting processes: acts of informing and forming. In: S Friedman (ed.) *The Reflecting Team in Action.* The Guilford Press, New York.

Balint M (1964) *The Doctor, His Patient and the Illness.* Pitman Medical, London, UK.

Banyard VL and Graham-Bermann SA (1993) Can women cope?: a gender analysis of theories of coping with stress. *Psychol Women Q.* 17: 303–18.

Bendelow G (1993) Pain perceptions, emotions and gender. *Sociol Health Illness.* 15: 273–94.

Berger SE (1996) *Horizontal Woman: the story of a body in exile.* Houghton Mifflin Company, Boston/New York.

Borkan J, Reis S, Hermoni D and Biderman A (1995) Talking about the pain: a patient-centered study of low back pain in primary care. *Soc Sci Med*. **40**: 977–88.

Eccleston C, De C Williams A and Stainton Rogers W (1997) Patients' and professionals' understandings of the causes of chronic pain: blame, responsibility and identity protection. *Soc Sci Med*. **5**: 699–709.

Gijsberg CM and Kolk AM (1997) Sex differences in physical symptoms: the contribution of symptom perception theory. *Soc Sci Med*. **45**: 231–46.

Jensen I, Nygren Å, Gamberale F, Goldie I and Westerholm P (1994) Coping with long-term musculoskeletal pain and its consequences: is gender a factor? *Pain*. **57**: 167–72.

Jensen MP, Turner JA, Romano JM and Karoly P (1991) Coping with chronic pain: a critical review of the literature. *Pain*. **47**: 249–83.

Johansson E (1998) *Beyond Frustration: understanding women with undefined musculoskeletal pain who consult primary care* (dissertation no. 550). Department of Family Medicine, Umeå University. Unpublished.

Johansson E, Hamberg K, Westman G and Lindgren G (1999) The meanings of pain: an exploration of women's descriptions of symptoms. *Soc Sci Med*. **48**: 1791–802.

Mechanic D (1995) Sociological dimensions of illness behavior. *Soc Sci Med*. **41**: 1207–16.

Penn P and Frankfurt M (1994) Creating a participant text: writing, multiple voices, narrative multiplicity. *Fam Process*. **33**: 217–31.

Raymond MC and Brown JB (2000) Experience of fibromyalgia: qualitative study. *Can Fam Physician*. **46**: 1100–6.

Stewart M, Brown JB, Weston WW *et al*. (1995) *Patient-Centered Medicine: transforming the clinical method*. Sage Publications, Thousand Oaks, CA.

Vygotsky L (1988) *Thought and Language*. MIT Press, Cambridge, UK.

4

Understanding the whole person

Judith Smith grew up with four younger siblings. Her mother died when she was 10, and she had to take care of the younger ones after her death. An uncle often came to visit the family, but Judith would stay away from the house when he arrived because he would always get very close to her. When she was 13, at a moment when Judith's father was out, her uncle started making sexual approaches to her. He said he would kill her if she told anybody about their 'little secret'. Even now, she has still not told her husband Greg.

She met Greg when she was 17 and got pregnant easily. Greg, a carpenter, is a pleasant man who spends most of his spare time with his buddies, repairing old wooden boats and sometimes having a few beers. He is eager for sex, but Judith's body no longer gives her any pleasure, only burdens. John, their oldest son, works at a factory and lives nearby with his wife, whom he recently married. Their daughter, Emmy, became a single mother at the age of 16 and works hard in a supermarket to have a decent income. Greg's mother suffers from progressive symptoms of Alzheimer's disease and needs more care every week. Last week, the neighbors found her walking in the street with no shoes on. Judith knows that she is the only one who is able to understand and take care of her mother-in-law, although the extra work makes her very tired.

Judith has several friends whom she sees now and then. They get together to share confidences and to enjoy each other's company and some sweet desserts without feeling guilty about the whipped cream and the calories. Judith started working at the hospital laundry many years ago, and she loves her work although it is monotonous and heavy. When she has been on vacation for a few days, she misses her co-workers, the coffee breaks and the jokes, although she does not miss her boss, who makes a pass at every woman employee whenever he gets the chance.

The second component of the patient-centered clinical model is an integrated understanding of the whole person, including the patient's individual development, family lifecycle and social context. Approaching these areas may enhance the physician's interaction with the patient, especially when the symptoms do not point to a clearly defined disease, or when the patient's response to an illness appears exaggerated or out of character. Issues in family life and worklife can provide explanations for mechanisms leading to pain, as well as being the context of living a life in pain. In this chapter, we shall explore the role of various family lifecycles on the background and context of living with pain, especially with regard to dysfunctional families where abuse occurs, as well as structural inequities giving rise to disempowerment and strain.

Family, work, health and rehabilitation for women in pain

Katarina Hamberg and Eva E Johansson

To gain a more comprehensive understanding of women patients with biomedically unexplained musculoskeletal pain, we conducted a research project where semi-structured interviews were used to explore the life situation of women with these symptoms. Qualitative analysis was performed to learn more about the meaning of activities and priorities in daily living (Hamberg *et al.*, 1997, 1999; Johansson *et al.*, 1997, 1999). Questions we posed were: What's it like at work? What are your aspirations for your work? What does employment mean to you? What's it like at home? What about conditions in the marital relationship? Can exploring the circumstances at home help us grasp the difficulties in the rehabilitation of women with myofascial pain?

Who were the women we talked with?

Twenty women between 21 and 61 years, sick-listed due to myofascial pain, participated. Careful investigation of their complaints showed no biomedical diagnosis that could fully explain their pain. All were employed, half of them full-time. The majority had limited education and physically demanding jobs with low income. Home-help, nursing assistant and cleaner were typical jobs. All but one of the women had children and all had been or were co-habiting with a man. Thirteen had prior experiences of divorce, two more divorced during the study and five entered new relationships.

The study was conducted in Sweden, where official policy since the 1970s has encouraged equality between women and men in all sectors of society. Gender-equality legislation now includes such reforms as parental leave for fathers as well as mothers and efforts to increase gender equality at the workplace. Eighty per cent of Swedish women between 20 and 64 years of age are in the labor force, and 64% of them have full-time jobs (Statistics Sweden, 1995). The state policy of gender equality and the effort to include the vast majority of all individuals in the workforce have made a strong impact on what it means to be a woman in Sweden. However, in everyday life, official policy on gender equality contrasts with more traditional attitudes toward femininity that uphold the notion of separate spheres for women and men, as well as the assumption that housework and childcare are women's duties.

Labor life: self-esteem and economic survival

The women all described what they expected from 'a good job': economic independence, stimulation and personal recognition. At the same time they described discrepancies between their aspirations and their actual working conditions. They questioned their expectations of worklife and lowered their hopes.

For these women it was hard to expect a job might enable them 'to manage on your own', and to become economically independent. Rather, many expressed that they had 'no chance to survive' on their wages. Although the security and routine of a steady job were desired, many had to accept temporary jobs. Young as well as old had not chosen a career, but taken whatever job that had come in their way, in order to 'earn a living'. They were now 'stuck' in jobs with limited economic prospects. Sofie, a 31-year-old cleaner, said:

'We were seven at home. I started working afternoons when I was 14 to support myself and get some of my own money. I have no educational ambitions. I'm not a climber. Not as long as I get along moneywise.'

The women also wanted a job to be 'varying', 'not too heavy', and to have 'a purposeful content':

'First of all, a job is an economic matter. But then, also a habit, and it should be fun. Getting out, meeting other people and having working mates.'

However, instead of stimulating social contacts, the majority described social tensions at their workplace, involving workplace reorganization, threat of redundancy and even bullying. One cleaner reported:

'If you're at work and maybe you say you are in pain, then you hear, "Who isn't?", all the time. It puts you in a bad mood . . . It's as if she wants to assert herself and make a fool of me in front of the others.'

A job was important for self-esteem: 'If you don't have a job you're nobody'. Some were proud to be industrious and described themselves as being always on-duty. Old as well as young expressed a wish to be needed by others at work; to be someone who is 'useful' and takes care of the little ones: 'I know I have a lot to give. I'm a good listener, I care for others, I stand by'.

Contrasting their dreams, the women had low-income jobs in fields threatened by redundancy, such as cleaning, care and service. Their partners also had low wages but usually earned a little more per month. Most of these women went unnoticed at their workplace and they expressed frustration with their lack of recognition despite steady attendance:

'I'm the kind that tries to please others. . . . One has to wait, to adjust, to be likeable and . . . damn it!'

Of course, there were examples of personal reinforcement at work. Often, however, it was only when a woman had been absent that she was noticed:

'The nurses said: "Oh wonderful that you're back. We haven't figured out how to use the sterilizing machine"'.

Regardless of age and years at work, these women did not identify with their actual profession, but rather with the tasks. The cleaner said, 'I do the cleaning', and the waitress, 'I work at a lunch bar'. The paid work was not their main source of self-esteem and identity.

Instead, the family was the main arena for both social and personal reinforcements, and family considerations had a strong impact on the organization and priorities of their paid work. Access to income, social contacts and personal development at work were balanced against childcare and other family responsibilities. The woman in the family was the one who arranged her life in order to take proper care of the children and despite work ambitions, she prioritized family commitments before paid work if those were in conflict. The mothers had made social arrangements in order to be available at home. They had chosen part-time jobs, working shifts and nights to piece together work and childcare. They were not 'too engaged' in the job, and not active in the trade union movement. By choosing unsociable working hours, however, they had to give up work aspirations, such as meeting people and gaining a 'working identity'.

Sharing family responsibilities and duties

What did the women tell us about their family life? What about the concrete division of unpaid work and activities; domestic duties, caring responsibilities and time for own activities?

With small variations, the women described themselves as being responsible for domestic duties such as cleaning, laundry, cooking and shopping. Their spouses contributed by taking responsibility for the car, the upkeep of the family home, and by being the 'handyman' in heavier duties:

> 'I'm responsible for the home and he is responsible for the car. We never thought about that.'

Most of the women, older as well as younger, carried or had carried the main part of the parenthood responsibilities. Whether or not the woman lived with the biological father of the children, the organization of the children's everyday life activities was, or had been, on her shoulders:

> 'I was alone with the kids during the week. He never took them to the day-care center, made food or anything like that. So when I divorced it made no difference.'

The women also perceived themselves as responsible for caring obligations toward close relationships, such as keeping in contact with sisters and brothers, being on hand for grandchildren and helping parents and aging relatives:

> 'My mother-in-law can no longer take care of herself. She forgets to eat and to keep herself tidy. She does not let anybody but me wash her up or help her in the bath.'

The women felt ashamed and guilty if they weren't effective and 'on hand' at home. Time for their own personal activities was a delicate issue, especially when the children were little and needed looking after. The women described tense discussions with their partners about responsibilities when they needed time for their own activities, such as physiotherapy or physical exercises:

> 'He looks after our son while I'm exercising. Well, we often argue about it, but he does do the baby-sitting anyway.'

The participants' instant explanations for why they carried the main burden of unpaid work while their spouses were expected to prioritize paid jobs were mainly superficial legitimizations, such as 'fair sharing' and 'best suited' or write-offs such as 'never thought of'. However, other motives also became obvious; they were striving for love and social acceptance and hoped to manage the family budget.

In the situation of chronic pain, the participant had difficulties managing the bulk of family duties. In her efforts to change the division of labor at home, it became obvious that to be worthy of love, the woman restricted what she negotiated. It was a big step to reduce the level of service, as it was a source of reinforcement and appreciation from her partner:

> 'He was not interested in my job ... he always appreciated me for being a good mother and an excellent cook. He told others that "my wife is a very good cook", and when he came home he might say "The table looks real nice".'

In cases of abuse, shame and fear restricted what the participants might discuss with their partners. A risky situation might arise if they did not carry out 'their' duties well enough:

> 'He once told me he could not love me as a woman because there was dust on the shelves and the floor.'

As described in Chapter 3, the pain often had consequences for the women's caring duties. When it was hard for them to live up to wishes and expectations, either from themselves or relatives, they felt ashamed and belittled. To be accepted in the eyes of others (relatives, friends and workmates) was important for the women. Value judgements, such as 'minding the children is a woman's concern' and 'family comes first', were mentioned in passing as matters of course or generally shared values.

When a woman was sick-listed she might need help and support from her husband and children with the domestic duties, but if she got help, she might hear that she had nothing to complain about, having such a nice family. A husband who shared domestic duties was regarded as a precious gift to the woman, who ought to be very grateful. The other side of the coin was that if a woman's family helped out with domestic tasks, she might not feel accepted as a good wife and mother. Likewise, in our clinical practice, during discussing with men and fathers it becomes obvious that norms about manliness frame their considerations. A male patient in his 40s told one of us that he used to draw the curtains when he cleaned the dishes, and another said that he did not tell his mates that he stayed away from football because he had to take care of his daughter. Instead, he excused his absence by referring to fever and illness. In this way, norms about 'womanliness', 'manliness' and what is appropriate for each sex to do create frames and guidelines for the organization of family life.

Efforts to manage the family budget could explain much of the unequal balance of domestic and parental responsibilities. All the participants had low incomes.

The man usually earned a little more, and the family economy required that he had a full-time paid job. Thus, the woman was the one who had to be flexible; she began to work nights or part-time to be able to take care of the children. Still, it was not economy alone that was crucial. In instances when the husband earned less or was even unemployed the woman still carried the main burden of unpaid work at home. Such contradictions led us to look further into negotiations and decision-making in the family.

How were decisions made at home?

According to gender theory, more consideration and importance in society is given to men than women (Candib, 1995; Connell, 1987). In our study, the women emphasized that in their marital relationships the needs of both parties were considered when decisions were made, and that they themselves made many decisions on behalf of the family. However, on a day-to-day basis, the women's decisions were adjusted to the unquestioned frames of a gender power structure.

The quotation below is typical of the way power and decision-making appeared in the study. Elsie did not see her husband as dominating, but interpreted within a gender perspective, the power structure in the relationship becomes obvious:

> **Elsie:** *I'm the one who decides. When there is a lot of money involved, we discuss it.*
> **Researcher:** *Would it be possible to get rid of the dog? I think that would be good because of your and your son's allergy.*
> **Elsie:** *Oh no, my husband would never allow that! Maybe I can make him accept that the new dog will sleep outdoors. Hunting is very important to him; I would not like to stop him from doing that.*

We do not have to distrust Elsie when she stated that she was the one who made decisions in her family. However, norms and values of womanliness and 'a woman worthy of love' implied an unspoken submissiveness that had an impact on how the division of duties, as well as decisions, were carried out. To strive for love also meant not to demand 'too much' from the man. To strive for social acceptance meant suppressing or adapting one's wishes if they did not fit into the gender norms.

Adjustment to a role of female subordination also characterized the women's efforts to manage the family budget. The husband was looked upon as the breadwinner, and more consideration was given to his paid work and career prospects, even if she earned more money. For example, Ruth was the one who managed to get steady jobs. Nevertheless, her husband's dream of a business of his own had preference over her wage-earning; when he moved, she moved with him, and she was the one who was responsible for the children:

> 'He said one day that he had bought a store in another town. I had a nice job ... but, well, we moved. But ... he did not make enough money. Then he bought another small firm and we moved again. Anyway, I took a job as a clerk and had a woman look after our baby ...'

Domestic abuse

The occurrence of violence and threats against women is an important aspect of the family context. Experiences of abuse were delicate matters to discuss, despite our efforts to create a close and intimate interview situation (Hamberg *et al.*, 1999). The women hesitated to speak about abuse and showed by sighing and pausing that it was hard for them. Still, we were struck by the fact that as many as 11 of the 20 participants described different experiences of violence or threats.

Ten had been abused by a former or present intimate partner. They described various kinds of physical violence – threats, fear – and needing to be constantly on guard. They underlined that threats were just as hard to survive as the physical violence:

> 'In the end, I was afraid all of the time. And then I had to accept it because it was always my fault, of course. .... You never got to say anything. Wasn't allowed to have my own opinions, because he saw them as insults. ... I wasn't allowed to vacuum, but the house had better be clean.... You never knew what you were supposed to do. Sometimes, he would kick me out of the bed in the middle of the night. Once, he jumped on me and grabbed me by the hair and pulled and banged my head against the floor and spat on me.'

The majority of the abused women described the abuse as one root of their pain. One had chronic sinusitis and facial pain which she described as a consequence of a severe battering. More commonly, tensions and anxiety due to fear and threats were given as causes of pain. Years after having left the abuser, some still referred to the violence as a cause of their present health problems:

> 'When I feel sick mentally, I get all tensed up and when I am tense my back hurts. .... The reason that I don't feel well nowadays has nothing to do with my daily life, but it's things that remind me of things that happened then ... And so, if you could only ... just erase them, everything but the last two years, then you'd have a pretty ideal life.'

Our results confirm previous research, further explored by Candib in the next part of this chapter, that in certain groups of women seeking healthcare, the occurrence of violence and threats is very high. Without stating anything about causality, our research shows that it is necessary to reflect on and ask about abuse in women patients suffering from chronic pain.

Coping with family commitments and rehabilitation programs

The women in our study primarily related their pain and need for rehabilitation to strains in their paid work. Family life was perceived as a private matter, outside the area of medical intervention. At the same time, in their narratives the women underlined the amount of work they had to do at home as an explanation for not complying with the rehabilitation plans or the doctor's advice. Family duties could show up as obstacles, e.g. in the use of sick leave and physiotherapy, and in discussions about alternative jobs.

The participants often found it difficult to use their sick leave for rest and treatment. Even when sick-listed, they still tried to uphold their part of the family duties. Some even felt stronger demands and thus tended to work more at home:

> 'Now that I'm sick-listed and at home, I have to see to it that the house is clean and the dishes are washed. It is different when one is working.'

On the other hand, a woman could also refer to the unpaid work at home as a reason for her need for sick leave. One woman asked for part-time sick leave because she was too tired to take care of her two children satisfactorily when she worked full-time. She had to get up early to take them to the day-care center, and she picked them up late in the evening.

In general, the participants expressed positive attitudes toward physiotherapy. However, their attitudes were inconsistent with the fact that they were often absent from training sessions and had difficulty following through with training programs at home. Various reasons why this was so were given, like 'I've never engaged in sports' or 'I'm too fat to undress in public baths'. Nonetheless, the difficulties were often related to family commitments. The time for physiotherapy had to fit in with family responsibilities. To choose a type of keep-fit exercise that they could bring the children to could be the only way for mothers with small children:

> 'I exercise by bicycling. Then my little son can come along – sitting behind me in the child seat.'

There were examples of women giving up the rehabilitation programs they were offered because they interfered with the organization of their family life. Elsie postponed her stay at the rehabilitation institute, which was located in another part of the country. It was hard for her husband to change his working hours in order to take care of the children. When at last she left for a four-week stay at the rehabilitation center, she had worked hard to fill the freezer with ready-to-eat, home-cooked food.

When Swedish patients suffer from CMP, the workplace is inspected to determine what can be done to ease the patient's physical and psychosocial strain at work. In this study, many of the women had physically demanding jobs, and there were examples of psychosocial strain, such as bullying and harassment, that made it necessary to initiate discussions at the workplace or plan for an alternative job or studies.

Often disregarded in rehabilitation is the emphasis many women place on an educational program or a job to be compatible with family life. These women claimed it was important that during further training they did not bring in less money to the household, and that when they took part in training courses, they could also take care of the family. Work or studies should not be located too far from home, nor should they infringe on their off-duty life, forcing them to be 'preoccupied by the job at home'. Carrying, as they did, the full parental responsibility, there were major problems interfering with their rehabilitation:

> ' I did not do so well at tests, it did not work … My daughter got whooping-cough for eight weeks and then my son got it, too. I had to stay at home with them.'

To enter a study program or start vocational training was a step that often implied a strain on family life. Studying might require a woman to focus more on her own needs and possibilities. Sometimes the economic power in the family very evidently affected her rehabilitation opportunities:

> 'I would never have been able to study unless they (the state welfare office) had let me study with a sickness benefit. My husband wouldn't have let me go.'

What did the woman do when commitments in the family obstructed her opportunities to participate in rehabilitation and to find new solutions for recovery or ways to cope with the pain? As a rule, the woman first presented the organization of her family life as self-evident and nothing worth talking about. She seemed satisfied, 'accepting the terms', not wanting to give up any chores. However, when the pain became long-term, she could not do as much domestic work as before and found herself in a situation with contradicting demands. As sick-listed, but without obvious signs of disease, she felt pressure from herself, her partner, children and friends to do more at home. On the other hand, the social insurance authorities and her doctor demanded rehabilitative activities or rest, and did not take into account her responsibilities at home. She was also tempted by rehabilitation opportunities such as training courses or jobs, but ran into difficulties 'fixing it all'.

Changing the patterns

Sofie, a 31-year-old cleaner, was married and had two pre-school children. She described her situation in the family as traditional and self-evident:

'It's my duty to run the household ... my opinion is that the women should take care of the children and not leave them at a daycare center ... He makes more money than I so if we disagree, his decision is final.'

However, because of her pain it was hard for her to do the main share of the housework. She questioned the terms and persuaded her husband to increase his involvement in the household:

'I made him do the washing today. I told him he only had to press that button. It was the first time in 10 years.'

At first, Sofie spoke about her responsibility toward the children and said it was impossible for her to take part in any of the training programs offered. Parallel with discussions with the physician about the conditions in the family, a process started in which Sofie began questioning both her ideas about child-rearing and aspects of the division of labor with which she was formerly satisfied. She discussed these issues with her husband and achieved several changes. He changed his working schedule in order to be able to look after the children while she went to physiotherapy. She started to study, in order to be able to get a less heavy and more stimulating job, and left the children at a childcare center.

For Sofie, this was a desired development which had been the result of some self-perception changes. She had come to the personal realization that a change was needed, acceptable and likely to be achieved. She needed to consider what consequences the changes might have on a personal, family and economic level. What would she gain and what might be lost? Could she rely on her husband to take care of the children? Could the family afford the costs of the childcare center? She needed to discuss such matters and test the arguments and effects of certain changes during the course of the rehabilitation.

Some women rejected proposals to alter the division of duties and priorities in the family even though they, like Sofie, might describe a very sex-segregated pattern.

Understanding the whole person then implied respecting the woman's perspective and trying to adapt the rehabilitation measures to what could be accomplished within the current family situation. In Elsie's case, rehabilitation had to fit in with the childcare situation because her husband did not take any responsibility for the childcare. To find a job for Elsie required flexibility on the part of the rehabilitation team, and a readiness to respect her viewpoint on the possibilities of changing the organization of her private life, as well as her preference for accepting the terms as they were.

However, there were situations where the participants' adherence to family commitments might be seen as a way of escaping what the rehabilitation measures required of them. Then it was important to continue the discussion about priorities and routines, trying to understand her reasons, finding out what the patient wanted and needed and, if possible, how to achieve that.

Those living with a man who threatened or abused them had narrow margins for changes in their private life. On the whole, they had no option other than to accept or leave. It was not until they had decided on leaving that they were able, or willing, to discuss their experiences in the marital relationship. Lena was married to a man who threatened her in various ways. While she was still married, she described her pain exclusively in relation to her paid job:

> 'The worst is the hurry and the stress. People are often sick and absent but we must do all the work anyway ... I have to stretch and reach out ... there is heavy lifting all the time.'

At the end of the study, Lena left her husband. Then she could speak about the situation she had been living in, and about her own ideas concerning the impact of her marriage on her pain:

> 'While we were living together ... When I was anxious I had a headache and shoulder pain. I knew exactly why. I worried about him ... He might stay away nights. He might come home drunk. It was not so bloody funny with him thudding about, falling on the bathroom floor, perhaps ...'

In the rehabilitation process, the divorce meant a new situation where it became easier to deal with family issues and to discuss ways to cope with the pain, although her pain persisted.

The marriage contract

Our study taught us that family considerations are not only of crucial importance to the patient's mode of action in order to recover or relieve the pain, but also to how a rehabilitation process can be outlined. To develop concepts that help physicians understand the whole person, and to grasp central aspects of family life more easily is of great importance to our discipline. Our contribution to this work is to summarize our knowledge about family conditions in the form of the 'marriage contract'.

Social science researchers have used the term 'marriage contract' to refer to ideas, patterns and frames that have an impact on the relations between men and women in society (Haavind, 1984; Pateman, 1988). The content of the contract varies between societies and is based on traditions and cultural norms about womanliness and manliness as well as laws. More recently the concept of 'gender order' has gained acceptance and more or less replaced the marriage contract as a broad concept focusing on relations between men and women on a societal level (Connell, 1987).

However, we found it useful to apply the concept of the marriage contract to conceptualize our findings about the women's family considerations. By 'marriage contract' we mean the habits, rules and agreements regulating who does what and what is proper behavior in a couple. Who takes responsibility for the children's school, health and peer problems? What chores have priority and on what grounds? What is more important, a new motor for the boat or a sewing machine? What can the woman do without putting her femininity in question? What can the man do and still be a 'real' man?

The marriage contract is usually not openly verbalized, but rather is subconscious and has developed gradually. It rests on traditions and culture in the society, but also on the individuals' wishes, interests, strengths and power. No signed paper exists; the contract is a theoretical concept. The appropriateness of the contract concept is most easily seen when habits and division of duties have to be changed. Then discussions and frustration occur. 'We always used to . . .'. In the consultation, the marriage contract is a useful tool when exploring the relation between an individual man and woman.

Figure 4.1 illustrates the marriage contract with three levels: the first is the concrete division of family duties, the second the motives for the priorities, and the third level the decision-making in the family. By exploring the patient's family life according to these three levels, it may be possible for the physician to grasp the frames and conditions of the private marital world. On each level it is possible to discuss priorities and options with the patient, opening up opportunities to find new ways to handle problems she might have run into in the situation of pain.

When the motives for division of responsibilities in the family are discussed during the encounter, the woman's own participation in creating her conditions can be illuminated. She becomes an actor who facilitates dialogue about changing patterns and habits, instead of the passive recipient of advice from the doctor. The marriage contract as a model with three levels may serve as a guide in the discussion. It leaves room for the individuality and variation that is necessary for it to work in consultations with different kinds of patients. After

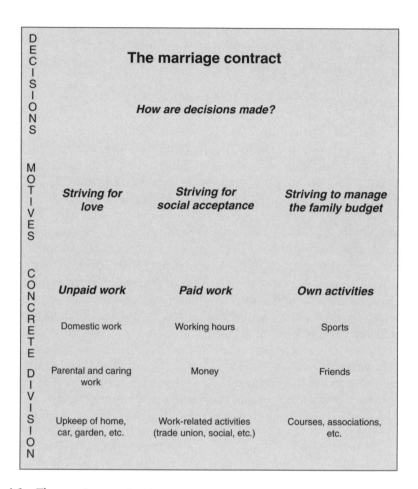

Figure 4.1 The marriage contract.

all, women are different; not all adjust to the same norms of womanliness. The marriage contract can also be applied as a guide in consultations with patients living in other circumstances than the studied women, e.g. men or women with more education or high-status jobs. To illustrate the usefulness of the marriage contract, the reader might reflect on her or his own private relations according to the marriage contract.

During office visits, it is necessary to make very specific inquiries into family life to receive relevant answers. Instead of asking in general terms about the situation at home, it is advisable to ask for descriptions of the division of duties and consequences of changes in the patterns in the family. Appropriate questions might be 'Could you tell me about the morning routines in your family?', 'What could be done to make housework easier for you?', and 'What would happen in your family if you were to go back to school?'. Hypothetical questions like 'If you had 1000 dollars, what would you do and why?' might also work as a start for discussions on priorities and needs. Thereafter the terms of the marriage contract become more visible, and the discussion of health, treatment and rehabilitation can continue from a shared understanding of the alternatives available to the woman.

> As a teenager, Judith dreamed of becoming a teacher. She enjoyed school and demonstrated talents for mathematics and English. However, she had a lot of work and responsibilities at home, caring for her younger siblings, and did not do that well at school. When she met Greg and became pregnant, there was no alternative except finding a job to earn money. The first years as a mother she worked part-time, in the evenings, in a bar. Then Greg took care of John while she was working. Later, she got the job at the laundry.
>
> Judith would have preferred to go to college and educate herself for a job that was not as physically demanding as her present one. The question is, however, who will pay the bills? Greg's income is not that big and she doesn't want to bother him with finances right now. He is saving all he possibly can to buy a better motor for the boat, and Judith thinks he deserves the joy of a faster boat. Some of his buddies even have new ones ... If Greg could only understand just a little of what it means to have pain, and maybe help her with the shopping or vacuuming, without her continuous nagging.
>
> Judith feels pressure from the physician to show more interest in the physiotherapy and rehabilitation discussions, but he does not realize how hard it is to go to the physiotherapist when one is ashamed of being overweight and does not have suitable clothes for training. It is such a long way to the training center, too, and the bus schedule is not convenient. Last time it took three hours to go for half an hour of physiotherapy, and when she finally arrived at Greg's mother's place, the 'old girl' had put her stockings in the hot oven and nearly set them on fire.
>
> It is not easy to discuss such matters with the doctor when he talks about the importance of physiotherapy and the need for her to change job. And, who would like to employ Judith Smith?

A painful life: between multiple layers of oppression

Lucy M Candib

Chronic pain occurs within a multilayered context: the person's family of origin, his or her current family, worklife, and culture. Within culture, we must include the understanding of pain proffered by the medical establishment as well as the legacy of meanings passed down to us through various cultural forms, such as art, literature, music and drama. Culture also includes the lens of ethnicity: the vision of pain and how one experiences and understands it within one's own ethnic group. Within culture are also deeply embedded our assumptions about gender, assumptions that shape our beliefs in how one should live and work, get sick and age. These assumptions shape what it means for a man or woman to have such pain that he or she is unable to carry out the roles that she/he believes culture holds to be his/her responsibility.

When we try to understand the whole person, we will see that the experience of oppression, personal or social, is both the backdrop and the foreground of chronic pain. The patient-centered model applied to chronic pain allows us to explore the experience of medically unexplained pain within the patient's context, where we will see that oppressive structures and relationships are typical.

Culture and ethnicity

The impact of chronic pain on the life course is deeply related to a person's culture of origin. Across different cultures, specific sociocultural factors come into play: values about work, religious beliefs, local community standards and economic issues, kinds of governmental and social support programs as well as type and availability of healthcare. Each of these factors affects how patients and their physicians might regard chronic pain within the specific cultural context. Ethnicity mediates the experience of chronic pain, with the intensity of the pain and expression of the pain varying significantly among ethnic groups. Within a given ethnic group, the strength of the patient's heritage moderates how much pain she/he feels and expresses and how much it interferes in daily life (Bates *et al.*, 1993). Even within a cohesive and homogeneous culture, regional and community differences in the understanding of pain mediate a person's specific experiences of chronic pain.

Recent immigrants who have significant stresses of migration, dislocation, language difficulties, problems gaining access to healthcare and low social status (regardless of their social class in their homeland) may have particular trouble with chronic pain problems and may have more features of depression. Those most disempowered – the less cultured, older and less educated – are more likely to present chronic somatic symptoms as manifestations of depression. Those who suffered specific experiences of physical and psychological trauma in the course of war, imprisonment and migration will present complex syndromes of chronic pain to practitioners who must be aware of both the personal and cultural backdrop to a given individual's constellation of symptoms.

Asian, Hispanic, African, Mediterranean and most recently Eastern European immigrants to Western Europe and North America frequently present undifferentiated chronic pain problems to primary care clinicians. In addressing these problems, we must take into account both the individual and family histories of trauma and loss prior to immigration, and also the loss and alienation inherent in migration itself, as well as the discrimination and, at times, frank racism that immigrants and refugees continue to experience.

Pain, family and gender

Family therapy approaches have rarely examined the gender of the patient, the gendered division of labor and emotional work in the family, or the timing of chronic pain in the individual or family lifecycle (*see* Hepworth, 1987; Payne and Norfleet, 1986; Violon, 1985). Instead of seeing the whole person within the family context, work on chronic pain and the family during the 1970s–1980s instead pathologized the patient and the family. Explanations typical of such thinking included that the patient came from a family of origin where someone else had chronic pain (Violon and Giurgea, 1984); family members may share an increased sensitivity to pain or increased tendency toward 'pain behavior'. Spouses of chronic pain patients have been found to be highly perfectionist, implying their involvement in family dysfunction (Hewitt *et al.*, 1995), and also very symptomatic (Shanfield *et al.*, 1979), raising the possibility that patients with chronic pain pick spouses with chronic pain. Thus, the patient's pain causes his/her partner to develop symptoms, or the pain arises because the family is dysfunctional; thus, pain either comes from the dysfunction or stabilizes it. In this way of thinking, pain is a way for the patient to avoid dealing with problems in the family.

Another explanation from family dynamic thinking is that the patient's current family responds to his/her pain in a way that reinforces the pain and keeps it going. This idea is based on a belief in family homeostasis, a notion that has been used to blame the family itself for the continuation of a problem; e.g. to hold women responsible for domestic violence (Candib, 1995). Continuing this line of reasoning, much research on chronic pain patients has identified pathology in the relationship between the spouses, for instance holding that a high degree of mutuality is associated with worse outcome: 'double the resistance to change' (Swanson and Maruta, 1980). The negative relationship of spouse behaviors, particularly solicitousness to patients' pain or expression of pain, has been studied repeatedly (Jamison and Virts, 1990; Romano *et al.*, 1995; Turk *et al.*, 1987). Non-dysfunctional families with chronic pain patients may have been less studied. Contrasting research suggests that patients who feel that their families are supportive actually do better and report fewer problems on follow-up than those who describe their families as non-supportive (Jamison and Virts, 1990). While in the 1990s family therapy approaches to patients with chronic pain moved beyond the assumption that the symptom plays a role for the family (Anderson and Goolishian, 1990), medical practice absorbed the ideas of family homeostasis and secondary gain as promoting chronic pain, and has been slow to move beyond them.

In general, family-oriented studies of chronic pain have not identified gender of the person with the chronic pain and gender of the caregiver as a relevant issue. In one study, when the chronic pain patients were men, the wives showed more depression and marital dissatisfaction compared to husbands whose wives were chronic pain patients (Romano *et al.*, 1989), suggesting that the spousal role for women as caregivers to a partner with chronic pain is more stressful. In another study of spouses of chronic pain patients, 10 out of 12 highly distressed spouses were women, yet the reason why women spouses might be more likely to feel so much physical, emotional and social distress in relation to their husband's chronic pain was unexplored (Rowat and Knafl, 1985). Such studies of spousal relationships are unable to arrive at a whole-person perspective on chronic pain.

In the 1990s, 'biological' explanations of chronic pain in families were in vogue: contemporary studies, as with mental illness, emphasize biological characteristics of organisms that feel more pain, including emphasizing genetic predisposition to chronic pain problems. Such sociobiological thinking regarding family patterning of illness can be used to blame the bearers by attributing the clustering to 'bad genes'. Such an approach leads to the 'family context' being actively reinterpreted as the 'genetic' context rather than the relational context. Again, the whole person disappears.

Abuse histories and dysfunctional families

Recent research shows that women with many unexplained physical symptoms (sometimes called somatization) are more likely to come from dysfunctional families. Women with somatization (defined as more than 13 unexplained somatic symptoms from the NIMH Diagnostic Interview Schedule) are more likely than other women patients in primary care settings to come from families of origin where they experienced physical and sexual abuse and where physical violence, alcohol and drug problems were characteristic (Dickinson *et al.*, 1999). Here, instead of viewing the dysfunction as a property of a homeostatic system, we can clarify that the specific dysfunction was abuse of power, against women and children, across generational lines. This gives us a different way to think about women and chronic pain. We can see that the distress of childhood is held over and translated into physical symptoms in the adult, perhaps by way of retained body memories of fear and pain.

A past history of sexual abuse is typical (although not invariably present) in the life experience of women with other medically unexplained disorders – chronic pelvic pain (Walker *et al.*, 1988), chronic gastrointestinal pain (Drossman *et al.*, 1990), as well as fibromyalgia (Boisset-Pioro *et al.*, 1995; Taylor *et al.*, 1995). Fibromyalgia patients have a higher rate of contact-type abuse than control patients and are more polysymptomatic than control patients without medical illness (Taylor *et al.*, 1995). When women fibromyalgia patients are compared with other women rheumatology patients as controls, they are found to have a higher frequency of childhood sexual abuse, more contact abuse, more physical abuse in childhood and adulthood and more combined physical and sexual abuse (Boisset-Pioro *et al.*, 1995).

These findings suggest that for some, but not all, patients with fibromyalgia, inflicted physical and sexual harm serves as a backdrop to a chronic pain problem. It would be an error of *post hoc propter hoc* to say that abuse is the cause of the medically undefined disorders, but it is clear that a history of abuse is present for more than half of patients suffering with these conditions, and may play a role in predisposing or sensitizing women to chronic pain.

The climate of threat involved in child and adult sexual abuse results in a state of hypervigilance that can be directly connected with musculoskeletal tension and inability to relax. Patients with fibromyalgia have been shown to demonstrate higher levels of hypervigilance (McDermid *et al.*, 1996) suggesting that this mechanism may be particularly relevant to patients whose chronic pain involves the musculoskeletal system. A past history of physical abuse leaves a legacy of physical pain and injury on the body, while ongoing physical abuse maintains physical pain syndromes, and threats of physical abuse, including stalking, make fear a constant companion for many women. Battered women who experience a variety of kinds of abuse (physical, sexual, verbal) frequently present to physicians with pain problems, but the basic problem of abuse may go unrecognized both because of physicians' reluctance to inquire into this area and because of patients' shame in revealing their abuse. After two years of in-depth interviews, eight of Hamberg and Johansson's 20 subjects, selected for their symptom of chronic pain, ultimately revealed ongoing abuse, while 11 acknowledged having been abused at some time. Thus, musculoskeletal pain in women may actually represent a physical expression of women's oppression within the family context – both the family of origin and the family of procreation (the current family).

The gendered division of labor

In contemporary Western society, many women are expected to work full-time, maintain a relationship, raise children, manage a household, handle the needs of both children and the older generation, perform according to the expectations of family and neighbors and not be affected by their condition of being out of power in the family and in the workplace. Even in the absence of abuse within their current family or family of origin, women may find themselves caught in gender-specific, illness-promoting patterns: caring dilemmas, taking responsibility for hopeless responsibilities, and self-blaming (Malterud, 1992).

As Hamberg and Johannsen point out in the first section of this chapter, women's musculoskeletal pain and rehabilitation occur within the context of the 'marriage contract', an unwritten agreement to uphold the gendered division of labor in the household that determines what is expected of the woman and what she expects of herself. Any change must take into consideration the woman's need to accept, negotiate, or break this contract (Hamberg *et al.*, 1997). Women internalize these gendered role expectations so that the inability to do ordinary household tasks becomes a source of further oppression from within: 'I don't have the satisfaction of a paycheck or of having done a job well. My home is my career, and I feel a failure at that. I feel like a burden to my husband and family, and I feel useless. Self-esteem is a real problem for me' (Kelley and Clifford, 1997).

The family as the context of excess caregiving

During the middle years, some women shoulder overwhelming responsibilities for several generations of the family or, like Judith Smith, for their husband's family. They are expected to 'be there' for children, grandchildren, parents, in-laws, and at times grandparents and aunts and uncles, at the same time as they presumably maintain a relationship with a spouse. Qualitative studies suggest that women with fibromyalgia are givers and nurturers who need to be fully in charge (Kelley and Clifford, 1997). Women's nurturant roles may, in fact, be a cause of increased physical and psychological distress: they may be unable to say 'no' to others' demands and can never stop and rest until someone else's needs are fulfilled. Caught in the 'sandwich' or 'squeezed' generation, many women find the enormity of the task to be 'just too much'. Their bodies give out. In Judith Smith's situation, the needs of her mother-in-law will continue to advance; at the same time, she must support her 16-year-old daughter and a new grandchild in the home. Demands from family will only escalate. At the same time, her abilities to meet her own needs for self-esteem flounder as she loses her work identity and, if her pain is severe enough, her ability to maintain her home as she would like.

Hamberg and Johanssen's study of Swedish working-class women with chronic pain reveals that these women actually view their worklife and work aspirations in terms of their childcare and family commitments (Johansson *et al.*, 1997). Chronic musculoskeletal pain in working-class women cannot be taken out of context: it must be interpreted within the framework of the gendered division of labor at home. This group assumed that paid work should not interfere with family life; they arranged their working conditions around childcare, and as a result, gave up the possibility of work aspirations and work identity. Chronic pain is likewise viewed in terms of this arrangement: 'I've tried to go in for my job, but . . . I couldn't stand it. I must have a life at home, too. I mean strength left over for the home duties'. Once sick-listed, these duties took on an even more heightened importance: 'Now that I'm sick-listed and at home, I have to see to it that the house is clean and the dishes are washed. It's different when one is working' (Johansson *et al.*, 1997). Chronic pain and illness does not relieve these women of the oppression of housework.

Although women like Judith Smith gain respect, self-esteem, and social support from paid employment, work can also be a liability and a source of chronic musculoskeletal pain. Research suggests that the combined effort to carry out paid work and domestic responsibilities produces an excessive burden on women. Among Swedish women who work more than 20 hours per week outside the home in jobs with low control, high home stress is predictive of psychosomatic strain. Psychosomatic strain was assessed by questions relating to fatigue, trouble 'getting going' in the morning, trouble falling asleep, and headaches (Hall, 1992). Exhaustion (defined as feeling exhausted more than three days a week at the end of the work day) is higher among women workers who do more domestic work at home, usually those with more children. When paid work and domestic work are added together, more than a third of women who work over 30 hours per week and do more than 21 hours of housework suffer from insomnia one or more times a week (Tierney *et al.*, 1990). Given the complex relationship between chronic pain and poor sleep, exhaustion and insomnia may be some of the physical stressors that bring on and perpetuate CMP.

Scandinavian studies show that unskilled women workers have the highest rate of sickness/absenteeism due to MSDs and that low-income women are more likely to be disabled by musculoskeletal ailments (Andersson *et al.*, 1993). Repetitive muscular tasks may create poorly understood overuse syndromes, also called repetitive or repetition strain injuries (RSI). The relationship between muscle tension, job stress and physical symptoms is complex yet real. Abusive and harassing work conditions and settings with low control and high demands create stress-related symptoms (Theorell *et al.*, 1991), yet physicians are unlikely to inquire into this area. Patients may be reluctant to acknowledge job stress or harassment for fear of being considered malingerers. Thus, physical and psychological job stress may be combined for working women who have no easy recourse for relief.

For many low-income women, their paid work replicates their domestic work: cleaning, wiping, lifting, washing, tending small children's needs (cleaning and caring). While they may withdraw from one set of low-status duties (paid work) because of pain, as Hamberg and Johansson's informants revealed, the other set does not go away and may even feel more obligatory because the woman is no longer employed outside the home. In low-income women (measured by low level of education in most studies), chronic pain is more highly associated with depression; such depression is also associated with unemployment in chronic pain patients (Averill *et al.*, 1996). Chronic pain, depression and unemployment may be connected for this group of women because there are fewer options for other employment besides jobs involving manual labor that they find unmanageable with chronic pain. Thus, various types of oppression characterize both the home and work settings of women with chronic pain.

Biographical disruption and the lack of recognition

Chronic pain inevitably alters and constrains the life course in ways that can be described as 'biographical disruption' (Bury, 1982). Initially, when symptoms are insidious, patients attempt to make sense out of the symptoms on their own. When they seek medical attention, they are seeking both legitimization of their suffering and the legitimacy of a label that justifies their need to limit activities, including taking time out to rest or to be off from work. Even patients with a 'legitimate' diagnosis like rheumatoid arthritis may find that employment settings and co-workers do not recognize their needs for a changed relationship to work (Bury, 1982). This is more likely to be true for working-class patients whose jobs offer less flexibility.

The first step of biographical disruption, thus, is the decision to seek help and look for a diagnosis.

> 'Clearly, where symptoms of a condition coincide with those widely distribu-
> ted in a population (in this case aches and pains) the processes of recognition
> and of legitimizing the illness are particularly problematic' (Bury, 1982).

For the patients with rheumatoid arthritis, their diagnosis 'marked a biographical shift from a perceived normal trajectory through relatively predictable chronological steps, to one fundamentally abnormal and inwardly damaging'. The final aspect of this step, referral and diagnosis, provided them with relief that their symptoms were justified and their behavior was warranted.

In contrast, patients suffering from the medically unexplained disorders do not achieve relief from a definite diagnosis, and remain in search of both a legitimate label and legitimization of their suffering. The lack of recognition by the medical establishment of these conditions creates an assault on a woman's credibility and her self-image as a hard worker, resulting in a 'pilgrimage' to find a practitioner who would believe her and establish her integrity (Reid *et al.*, 1991). Thus, the search for diagnosis and treatment of pain can in itself become an organizing feature of a person's life, such that previous interests and activities fall by the wayside in the relentless pursuit of relief. Particularly people whose diagnoses lack external structural validation – like RSI, TMJ (temporo-mandibular joint syndrome) or fibromyalgia – may trudge ceaselessly from one practitioner to another for validation. One TMJ sufferer described that he was ' "on the sidelines observing life go by, not really participating" while he continues the seemingly never-ending search for an answer' (Garro, 1994).

Chronic pain requires a person to rethink their whole biography, life trajectory and self-concept, based on the diagnosis or the search for a diagnosis. In this phase, people try to fit their illness into their lives and attribute it with some meaning (a shock, an assault, etc.) and try to explain why it happened to them in particular. The last step in biographical disruption involves the changing connection to social relationships based on the effect of illness (Bury, 1982). Some people with medically unexplained disorders use the invisibility of their condition to keep up appearances as long as possible. For others, the invisibility casts doubt on the legitimacy of their suffering and results in social stigma, isolation and withdrawal (Schlesinger, 1993). With medical experts themselves in disarray about the organicity (and thus legitimacy) of fibromyalgia and myofascial pain syndromes, it is not surprising that the families, friends and co-workers of patients with these diagnoses are inconsistent in their response to the patients' suffering.

Even people who persevere against the pain find they have little energy left for social activities and may refuse invitations in order not to disappoint others or be considered 'unreliable'. Some chronic pain sufferers switch to less demanding jobs or avoid career advancement opportunities in order not to risk their precarious health by preventing avoidable stress (Garro, 1994). Others may leave work entirely and seek complete disability. Other people may put their entire life on hold, as did this 23-year-old woman, Theresa, in Garro's study of TMJ patients:

> 'Right now my goal is getting rid of the pain before I can get on with my life ... you know, going back to school, getting married, having children even, having a career, doing, you know, the things I want to do with my life' (1994).

Finally, people with chronic pain conditions may have to relinquish their future and give up their dreams and aspirations; this acceptance of limitations is hard:

> 'It was a difficult period before one had accepted that it would stay like this – pain all the time ... and then you felt that "I will never be able to do these

things in my life. I will never be able to experience what I have not done now"
... It feels like a barrier for the rest of life then ...' (Henriksson, 1995).

Growth and empowering experiences can occasionally arise from the constraints brought about by chronic pain. Garro reports that a few TMJ sufferers used the opportunity to recognize that their priorities had been misguided and that they needed to change their lives. In other words, they concluded that the body was telling the mind something it could not grasp for itself. Another narrator expands on this: 'Pain may bring us to an authentic recognition of our own limitations and possibilities ... it may serve as a catalyst for much needed changes in our lives' (Bendelow and Williams, 1995). Here is a fibromyalgia patient with a similar recognition: 'Are we so indispensable that the world will stop because we are sick? Our families can still function without us taking full charge. Maybe now I can get down from the pedestal I thought I was on ... I have had to learn to ask for help, and my family has been very supportive. My attitude has changed recently, and I can accept their help and be grateful for it' (Kelley and Clifford, 1997). While none of these patients would have chosen a life of chronic pain, a few have learned to use the constraints of illness to transform their lives for the better.

Chronic pain and psychiatric illness

A complex relationship exists between medically unexplained disorders and psychiatric illness. Fibromyalgia patients, compared with matched rheumatoid arthritis patients, are more likely to meet criteria for depression and anxiety, and are more likely to have had troublesome factors in their childhood history (poor living conditions, separation from family, loss of parents and family violence) (Schuessler and Konermann, 1993). Higher background rates of violence and victimization among patients with somatization and fibromyalgia make it unsurprising to find a higher frequency of depression and anxiety. These conditions are not the equivalent of depression and/or anxiety, however, nor do they respond to isolated psychiatric treatment. The chronic pain syndromes of fibromyalgia, myofascial pain, TMJ, RSI and chronic pelvic pain all have a symptomatology of their own. The suffering resultant from the conditions themselves and their struggle to gain recognition for their suffering may lead to the development of depression.

Receiving a psychiatric diagnosis may in itself be oppressive. Despite the frequent co-occurrence of depression and anxiety with chronic pain problems, receiving a psychiatric diagnosis is not necessarily therapeutic for patients with medically unexplained disorders, and they may experience any psychiatric diagnosis connected with their chronic pain problems as dismissive and denigrating.

RSI patients found it impossible to acknowledge any stressors in their illness because it would have seemed tantamount to agreeing to a psychogenic etiology of their pain problem (Reid *et al.*, 1991). In general, chronic pain patients fear being classified as mentally ill because it would mean that their disorder was 'not real' (Johansson *et al.*, 1996; Reid *et al.*, 1991). The stigma connected with psychiatric diagnosis in some countries may be sufficient for both doctors and patients to avoid such diagnostic labels because of fear of the possible ramifications should a psychiatric diagnosis become attached to their permanent medical record, or should they be labeled as mentally ill in their search for governmentally sanctioned disability.

On the other hand, avoiding a diagnosis of depression can mean withholding potentially useful treatment from that group of patients who might benefit from pharmacotherapy and psychotherapy. For those chronic pain patients who meet the criteria for somatization, a careful review of past history may reveal a strong history of physical and sexual abuse in up to two-thirds of the group; these patients may additionally be suffering from PTSD or complex PTSD (Dickinson *et al.*, 1998). They are harmed by exhaustive and invasive medical workups and can benefit from treatment aimed at these conditions. Until recently, their symptoms were not understood as a reflection of the physical and sexual trauma they endured at the hands of family members.

Medical disempowerment of patients with chronic pain

Chronic pain patients are acutely aware of the importance of the biological discourse in medicine; they know that only biomedical, physiological diagnoses are considered legitimate and that pain that is 'invisible' – e.g. does not show up on tests – lacks legitimacy. Having medical providers think that their pain is a psychiatric illness is, to chronic pain sufferers, a form of oppression; they feel that they are not being taken seriously. Patients with fibromyalgia don't want to be labeled as hypochondriacs or malingerers but want to be understood and to have their experience of pain recognized as valid. Patients in safe interview settings acknowledge their experiences of not being believed by doctors and of not trusting the doctors in response. They use a variety of strategies to get the doctor to pay attention to them rather than write them off, as suggested by the patient who said:

> 'I've been crying my way through the medical service ... If I hadn't ... not one would have taken care of me ... It was thanks to my continual asking' (Johansson *et al.*, 1996).

The patient seeks help for chronic pain within the framework of the marked asymmetry of the doctor–patient relationship in which the doctor's role is stereotypically male, even if it is occupied by a female physician. The expectations of the social, economic and healthcare systems are that the woman's ailments are not to be taken seriously. Some women patients' response to this hierarchical arrangement is to enter into help-seeking by engaging in strategies that fit within stereotypical female roles, including being 'under a doctor' (Johansson *et al.*, 1996). Doctors, as well, behave according to gender-based assumptions. Doctors' recommendations for rest and activity restriction are biased by patient gender; medical providers steer women toward socially prescribed gender roles – housework and homemaking (Safran *et al.*, 1997). Analysis of the medical discourse of encounters with women shows that doctors tend to marginalize important contextual issues that contribute to women's distress and remain uncritical about the social problems that women face (Borges and Waitzkin, 1995). How much more must this bias be at work when the patient brings a problem of chronic pain that the frustrated physician can neither diagnose definitively nor treat effectively.

The primary care clinician, be they internist, family doctor or general practitioner, inevitably plays a role in social control. Patients must be referred for rehabilitation or certified for disability. Doctors have to take a stand on the legitimacy of the patient's complaint and at times throw their weight behind a patient's case in order to gain sick benefits, reduced responsibilities or disability. Although social problems have increasingly become 'medicalized', the medical care system is reluctant to acknowledge the social control function that doctors and medicine play in patients' lives and in society in general. One form of this control is to identify the patient as the problem. Professionals are insistent that they themselves are not to be blamed for the occurrence or persistence of the pain (Eccleston *et al.*, 1997). Instead, patients who seek help in pain clinics may find themselves pathologized. Pain management seminars for professionals and pain control centers define the chronic pain patient as deviant:

> 'Although the technical literature on chronic pain patients describes this population in amoral, psychologistic and psychoanalytical terms, the centrality of the problem-patient issue in everyday pain care management is conducive to the cognitive framing of these patients as members of a morally stigmatized, deviant population. The role of the pain worker, therefore, may be best viewed as that of an agent of social control' (Kotarba and Seidel, 1984).

Countering oppression: narratives

An alternative to medicalizing chronic pain, which removes it from the patient's life experience, is to find a way for the patient to situate her symptoms within her own life context. Narrative work offers both a clinical and research approach to such a contextual view of the patient with chronic pain. Qualitative research devoted to collecting and analyzing narratives has greatly enriched our understanding of the whole person suffering (Garro, 1994; Kelley and Clifford, 1997; Reid *et al.*, 1991; Schlesinger, 1993, 1996). Narratives collected over a long period of time may allow the gradual emergence of more sensitive issues, such as a personal history of sexual abuse or battering that may not come out during a one-time interview with a previously unknown researcher (Johansson *et al.*, 1996, 1997). On the other hand, the anonymity of the research interview may allow narratives to emerge about experiences with the medical care system that would not be told immediately to the physician.

Narratives can enable us to recognize in an experiential way the themes of loss of both independence and of relationships, and often loss of validation by family, work, friends and healthcare providers for patients suffering from medically undefined disorders. Through narratives, we can come to understand how not only the structural and functional aspects of lives are changed by chronic pain, but also how intimacy and relationships are affected. The challenge of maintaining a relationship with a partner in the face of chronic pain pushes some relationships to a deeper level and others to fall apart (Schlesinger, 1996). These understandings about the meaning and effects of chronic pain on the lives of patients can liberate healthcare professionals from the prejudicial constraints of the medical viewpoint. When healthcare providers can come to an agreement with patients about the nature of their health problem, the possibility of a better outcome is enhanced (Bass *et al.*, 1986).

The narrative approach can also be liberating for patients themselves. Stories can be collected in ways that allow others with similar symptoms to share their history and validate each other's experiences. Both self-help and therapeutic groups may offer this possibility to people with medically undefined disorders. Patients can also be encouraged to tell their stories in the form of written narratives. One participant in a therapeutic group that used written narratives gives this account:

> 'Fibromyalgia has made me more balanced. I consider myself a nurturer and giver, but what if everyone was the same? There need to be people who want to be nurtured, too. Perhaps fibromyalgia has helped me be a person who can allow others to nurture me sometimes and help others learn the skills required to be a giver' (Kelley and Clifford, 1997).

Some narratives are not easily accessible in memory; some are too awful to tell. Former prisoners of war, torture survivors, ritual abuse and incest survivors, all may have stories that they can only tell in bits and pieces, if at all. The clinical setting is not suited to the revelation of atrocities, and most clinicians in primary care are not prepared for this work. Nevertheless, patients with these experiences are in our examining rooms every day. Many traumatized patients suffer from chronic pain syndromes directly or indirectly related to the violence they experienced, but they may not be able to make any conscious connection between their pain and the victimization. Using narrative to see themselves as whole persons with coherent life stories is impossible because the story is not coherent, and they are not able to hold all the parts of themselves together as whole persons.

Individual and group psychotherapeutic settings are under study as safe places where the 'terrible narrative' can be 'returned to consciousness, expressed explicitly and coherently, and worked through in a supportive context' (Waitzkin and Magaña, 1997). The proliferation of physical and psychological symptoms of patients who are trauma survivors reveal the extreme end of the mind–body response to violence, victimization and oppression. To a lesser extent, patients with medically unexplained conditions are survivors of a variety of kinds of oppression, often including family and sexual violence. We should not be surprised to find their narratives troublesome to hear. Yet it is exactly bearing witness to those testimonies that offers some promise of acceptance and recognition, if not healing, for patients with conditions for which we have no answers.

> Judith Smith is a working-class woman whose life has been characterized by hard work ever since her mother's early death left her in charge of four younger siblings at the age of 10. Like other girls unprotected by a strong maternal caregiver, Judith was sexually abused by a male family member during her adolescence under threats so powerful and so shameful that she has never even told her husband about the abuse. Her marriage is characterized by a strongly gendered division of labor, and heavy caregiving commitments to both the older and the younger generation.
>
> Her work is heavy manual labor in a sexually harassing setting that does, however, provide her with a source of pride as a worker as well as social support and friendship. During the many years of physically exhausting manual labor combined with excessive caregiving responsibilities, Judith has not taken much pleasure for herself; indeed, the idea is foreign to her. She is not consciously aware of how gendered forms of oppression have limited her ability to care for herself since childhood nor how they continue to shape her domestic and occupational responsibilities. Class oppression – manual labor with its limited rewards and its physical toll – and gender oppression, including sexual abuse, sexual harassment and sharply demarcated gender roles, form the backdrop for Judith's current symptoms.
>
> Throughout her life, even in the present, Judith has not had control over men's use of and access to her body, and now that body is the medium of her suffering. Even her relationship with her trusted physician, to whom she turns for help, is sharply characterized by gender hierarchy. The usual

power difference between Judith and her doctor is now exacerbated by her supplicant role as a sufferer of chronic pain. Though Judith has found ways to take pride and enjoyment in parts of her life, oppressive relations have characterized every area of her life. Chronic pain can be the body's way of expressing and responding to the multiple layers of oppression.

References

Anderson H and Goolishian HA (1990) Chronic pain: the family's role in the treatment program. *Houston Med.* **6**: 104–10.

Andersson HI, Ejlertsson G, Leden I and Rosenberg C (1993) Chronic pain in a geographically defined general population: studies of differences in age, gender, social class and pain localization. *Clin J Pain.* **9**: 174–82.

Averill PM, Novy DM, Nelson DV and Berry LA (1996) Correlates of depression in chronic pain patients: a comprehensive examination. *Pain.* **65**: 93–100.

Bass MJ, Buck C, Turner L *et al.* (1986) The physician's actions and the outcome of illness in family practice. *J Fam Pract.* **23**(1): 43–7.

Bates MS, Edwards WT and Anderson KO (1993) Ethnocultural influences on variation in chronic pain perception. *Pain.* **52**: 101–12.

Bendelow GA and Williams SJ (1995) Transcending the dualisms: towards a sociology of pain. *Sociol Health Illness.* **17**: 139–65.

Boisset-Pioro MH, Esdaile JM and Fitzcharles M-A (1995) Sexual and physical abuse in women with fibromyalgia syndrome. *Arthritis Rheum.* **38**: 235–41.

Borges S and Waitzkin H (1995) Women's narratives in primary care medical encounters. *Women Health.* **23**: 29–56.

Bury M (1982) Chronic illness as biographical disruption. *Sociol Health Illness.* **1**: 167–82.

Candib LM (1995) *Medicine and the Family: a feminist perspective.* Basic Books, New York.

Connell RW (1987) *Gender and Power* (6e). Polity Press, Cambridge.

Dickinson LM, deGruy FV, Dickinson WP and Candib LM (1998) Complex PTSD: evidence from the primary care setting. *Gen Hosp Psychiatry.* **20**: 1–11.

Dickinson LM, deGruy FV, Dickinson WP and Candib LM (1999) Health-related quality of life and symptom profiles of female survivors of sexual abuse in primary care. *Arch Fam Med.* **8**: 35–43.

Drossman DA, Lesserman J, Nachman G *et al.* (1990) Sexual and physical abuse in women with functional or organic gastrointestinal disorders. *Ann Intern Med.* **113**: 828–33.

Eccleston C, de C Williams AC and Rogers WS (1997) Patients' and professionals' understandings of the causes of chronic pain: blame, responsibility and identity protection. *Soc Sci Med.* **45**: 699–709.

Garro L (1994) Narrative representations of chronic illness experience: cultural models of illness, mind, and bodies in stories concerning the temporomandibular joint (TMJ). *Soc Sci Med.* **38**: 775–88.

Haavind H (1984) Love and power in marriage. In: H Holter (ed.) *Patriarchy in a Welfare Society.* Columbia University Press, New York.

Hall EM (1992) Double exposure: the combined impact of the home and work environments on psychosomatic strain in Swedish women and men. *Int J Health Serv.* **22**: 239–60.

Hamberg K, Johansson EE, Lindgren G and Westman G (1997) The impact of marital relationship on the rehabilitation process of women with long-term musculoskeletal disorders. *Scand J Soc Med.* **25**(1): 17–25.

Hamberg K, Johansson EE and Lindgren G (1999) 'I was always on guard': an exploration of woman abuse in a group of women with musculoskeletal pain. *Fam Pract.* **16**(3): 238–44.

Henriksson CM (1995) Living with continuous muscular pain: patient perspectives. Part I: encounters and consequences. *Scand J Caring Sci.* **9**: 67–76.

Hepworth J (1987) Families and chronic pain. In: D Rosenthal (ed.) *Families in Stress.* Aspen, Rockville, MD.

Hewitt PL, Flett GL and Mikail SF (1995) Perfectionism and relationship adjustment in pain patients and their spouses. *J Fam Psychol.* **9**: 335–47.

Jamison RN and Virts KL (1990) The influence of family support on chronic pain. *Behav Res Therapy.* **28**: 283–7.

Johansson EE, Hamberg K, Lindgren G and Westman G (1996) 'I've been crying my way': qualitative analysis of a group of female patients' consultation experiences. *Fam Pract.* **13**: 498–503.

Johansson EE, Hamberg K, Lindgren G and Westman G (1997) 'How could I even think of a job?': ambiguities in working life in a group of female patients with undefined musculoskeletal pain. *Scand J Prim Health Care.* **15**(4): 169–74.

Johansson EE, Hamberg K, Westman G and Lindgren G (1999) The meanings of pain: a qualitative exploration of symptom descriptions in a group of female patients with long-term musculoskeletal disorders. *Soc Sci Med.* **48**: 1791–802.

Kelley P and Clifford P (1997) Coping with chronic pain: assessing narrative approaches. *Soc Work.* **42**: 266–77.

Kotarba JA and Seidel JV (1984) Managing the problem pain patient: compliance or social control? *Soc Sci Med.* **19**(12): 1393–400.

Malterud K (1992) Women's undefined disorders: a challenge for clinical communication. *Fam Pract.* **9**: 299–303.

McDermid AJ, Rollman GB and McCain GA (1996) Generalized hypervigilance in fibromyalgia: evidence of perceptual amplification. *Pain.* **66**: 133–44.

Pateman C (1988) *The Sexual Contract*. Polity Press, Cambridge.

Payne B and Norfleet MA (1986) Chronic pain and the family: a review. *Pain*. **26**: 1–22.

Reid J, Ewan C and Lowa E (1991) Pilgrimage of pain: the illness experiences of women with repetition strain injury and the search for credibility. *Soc Sci Med*. **32**: 601–12.

Romano JM, Turner JA and Clancy SL (1989) Sex differences in the relationship of pain patient dysfunction to spouse adjustment. *Pain*. **39**: 289–95.

Romano JM, Turner JA, Jensen MP *et al.* (1995) Chronic pain patient–spouse behavioral interactions predict patient disability. *Pain*. **63**: 353–60.

Rowat KM and Knafl KA (1985) Living with chronic pain: the spouse's perspective. *Pain*. **23**(3): 259–71.

Safran DG, Rogers WH, Tarlov AR, McHorney CA and Ware JE (1997) Gender differences in medical treatment: the case of physician-prescribed activity restrictions. *Soc Sci Med*. **45**: 711–22.

Schlesinger L (1993) *Pain, Pain Management and Invisibility: research in the sociology of healthcare*. JAI Press, Greenwich, CT.

Schlesinger L (1996) Chronic pain, intimacy and sexuality: a qualitative study of women who live with pain. *J Sex Res*. **33**: 249–56.

Schuessler G and Konermann J (1993) Psychosomatic aspects of primary fibromyalgia syndrome. In: S Jacobsen, B Danneskiold-Samse and B Lund (eds) *Musculoskeletal Pain, Myofascial Pain Syndrome and the Fibromyalgia Syndrome*. Haworth Medical Press, New York.

Shanfield SB, Heiman EM, Cope N and Jones JR (1979) Pain and the marital relationship: psychiatric distress. *Pain*. **7**: 343–51.

Statistics Sweden (1995) *Women and Men in Sweden*. Gender Statistics Unit, Stockholm, Sweden.

Swanson DW and Maruta T (1980) The family's viewpoint of chronic pain. *Pain*. **8**: 163–6.

Taylor ML, Trotter DR and Csuka ME (1995) The prevalence of sexual abuse in women with fibromyalgia. *Arthritis Rheum*. **38**: 229–34.

Theorell T, Harms-Ringdahl K, Ahlberg-Hultén G and Westin B (1991) Psychosocial job factors and symptoms from the locomotor system: a multicausal analysis. *Scand J Rehabil Med*. **23**: 165–73.

Tierney D, Romito P and Messing K (1990) She ate not the bread of idleness: exhaustion is related to domestic and salaried working conditions among 539 Quebec hospital workers. *Women Health*. **16**: 21–42.

Turk DC, Flor H and Rudy TE (1987) Pain and families: I. Etiology, maintenance and psychosocial impact. *Pain*. **30**: 3–27.

Violon A (1985) Family etiology of chronic pain. *Int J Fam Therapy*. **7**: 235–46.

Violon A and Giurgea D (1984) Familial models for chronic pain. *Pain*. **18**: 199–203.

Waitzkin H and Magaña H (1997) The black box in somatization: unexplained physical symptoms, culture and narratives of trauma. *Soc Sci Med.* **45**: 811–25.

Walker E, Katon W, Harrop-Griffiths J *et al.* (1988) Relationship of chronic pelvic pain to psychiatric diagnoses and childhood sexual abuse. *Am J Psychiatry.* **145**: 75–80.

5

The patient–clinician relationship

Judith Smith has had the same physician, Dr Roger Jamesson, for nine years now. Although she is not always satisfied with his listening abilities and his recommendations, she likes him. She cannot stand the thought of having to repeat this long story of hers to a new physician. Judith always hopes for cure, and she often comes to her physicians with suggestions about investigations and treatment programs that she has seen on TV, or her friends have recommended. However, she finds her physician quite reluctant on matters he did not initiate himself. Sometimes she feels that he blames her for having pain because she is not able to rest or exercise as he told her.

Sometimes when the pain is terrible, Judith hates the pain, her painkillers and her physician who is not able to provide any sort of relief. She even screamed at him some months ago that he would never be able to understand how terribly her muscles were aching. Afterwards, she regretted this outburst deeply and sent him a bunch of flowers to apologize.

Dr Jamesson admits he is tired of hearing the same story from Judith every time, knowing that there is nothing he can do. He believes that she is more depressed than she will ever admit, and cannot understand why she doesn't want antidepressants. When Judith is on his list of appointments, he knows that the day in the office will be delayed. However, he feels that it is his duty to be there for her, and hopes for some new and magical remedies to change their relationship.

The fifth component of the patient-centered clinical model is conscious attention to enhancing the patient–clinician relationship. Long-term illness bears the potential of placing immense strain on patient as well as clinician, but may also comprise mutual trust and satisfaction. In this chapter, we shall explore expectations, experiences, challenges and rewards in the patient–clinician relationship with patients suffering from CMP. Pearls and pitfalls on the long road where suffering must be lived and witnessed will be discussed, focusing on potentials and limitations of the physician's role. We shall look closely at how things may go wrong. We will then examine empowering approaches intended to accommodate the reality of feelings and despair, aiming for hope and long-term recovery by supporting the patient as a resource.

Difficult patient or difficult relationships: when things go wrong

Katarina Hamberg and Eva E Johansson

Despite the high aspirations we have of listening and understanding, just as Dr Jamesson and many other physicians have found, some consultations end with feelings of failure and frustration. These encounters have often been with patients such as Judith Smith who suffer from chronic pain and widespread MSDs.

The patient's symptom(s) presentation is usually the starting point of the encounter. On the basis of what physicians see and hear during the history-taking process, the traditional disease-centered consultation will proceed with a physical examination, laboratory tests and perhaps other investigations before we try to summarize a diagnosis and a management plan. Sometimes, though, physicians get lost in complex consultations. A frequent reason for frustration and perceived failure is that the physician never finds out why the patient came in the first place, cannot grasp the patient's problem and feels disappointed.

Which patients are perceived as difficult?

When the consultation is confusing, the physician may perceive the patient as 'difficult'. However, no association is found between perceived difficulty and common medical disorders, such as hypertension, cardiac disease, arthritis, diabetes and cancer. Difficult patients suffer from functional disorders, such as irritable bowel, tension headache and fibromyalgia (Hahn *et al.*, 1996). Furthermore, encounters concerning musculoskeletal pain problems result in less 'shared understanding', and more negative feelings than consultations in general. Unexplained symptoms and experiences are frustrating for the physician as well as for the patient. This may often lead to diverging talk, questions and opinions. Patients using medical language and suggesting self-diagnoses might lead the healthcare provider to categorize them as less likely to comply with treatment, and more likely to pose difficult management problems and to take up a lot of time.

Schwenk *et al.* (1989) identified two main factors affecting the physician's perceptions of a difficult patient: first, the medical uncertainty with vague, difficult-to-describe, undifferentiated medical problems, and second, interpersonal difficulty. Difficult patients are often described as demanding or manipulative. According to our own experiences, we would say that difficult patients are pointed out at medical school. Functional disorders that display themselves as illness in everyday life, and not as clearcut diseases within the biological body, are dealt with as anomalies. Thereby we, as physicians, are not trained to manage these problems although they are common conditions in our practices. Of course, problems are presented that cannot be solved by the physician, but the sources of frustration can be related to aspects of the healthcare system, communication difficulties or even personal issues from the physician's own life. The physician might feel that stalemate has been reached, or may be afraid of opening up 'Pandora's box' and thus being overwhelmed by the problem.

In difficult and awkward consultations, an instant reaction might be to blame the individual patient. To reach beyond the frustration, it is, nonetheless, necessary to consider how the physician could contribute to improving the consultation.

Meetings between experts

As patient adherence, healthcare utilization and improved health depend on patients' satisfaction with the consultations, it is certainly worthwhile to try to make it optimal. Research on the consultation has focused on how to improve the patient–clinician relationship. According to Pendleton, the desired outcome of a consultation is a shared understanding of the problem (Pendleton *et al.*, 1984). To achieve this, a patient-centered approach is required, emphasizing the patient's life situation, expectations and feelings.

Two persons and two world perspectives meet in the examining room. The physician is the medical expert and the patient the expert on her perceptions, feelings and fears. The physician's task is to explore both the disease and the patient's illness experiences within the context of her life setting with family, work, worries and beliefs. One problem in the consultation certainly lies in whether patient and physician talk about the same things and share the same interpretative framework and conceptual worlds. The patient–clinician interaction includes a selection process in what we say, hear and understand, and in what the patients tell and the physicians take notice of (Hamberg and Johansson, 1999; Johansson *et al.*, 1996; Salmon and May, 1995).

Most research on patient satisfaction and consultation interaction focuses on the two individuals, their skills and style in communication, but often disregards such contextual background factors as gender, socioeconomic status and power, as discussed in Chapter 4. Noteworthy is that women constitute the majority of chronic pain patients as well as 'difficult patients' (Schwenk *et al.*, 1989). Since we emphasize the significance of gender and power in the patient–physician relationship, we shall implement a gender perspective in the patient-centered clinical method in this chapter.

Experiencing mutual distrust

We conducted a qualitative interview study to learn more about what women patients with chronic pain expect and experience, and how they act when they consult a physician. The 20 women interviewed presented ample experiences of utilizing medical service. While seeking help for chronic or recurrent pain problems, they described many instances of feeling disappointed and frustrated with the medical system.

All of the women gave examples of distrust in the consultation; feeling both distrusted and mistrusting of their physicians. They said they 'wanted a diagnosis', and if no bodily pathology was found, they feared being judged as mentally ill or as malingering and troublesome. They described being in a vulnerable position. As patients, they were exposed to the physician's ability to define the illness and to decide about treatment measures, such as prescriptions, referrals and certificates. If they took part in the medical dialogue or suggested a diagnosis or requested certain investigations, the physician might turn hostile. This was the way Ellinor expressed how she felt ignored, disregarded, and rejected in the consultation:

> '. . . When the physician arrived, he had a ready-made diagnosis and didn't listen to what I said. I talked to him about my back pain and how I perceive that the trouble in my feet and legs is connected with the spine. He said that was pure rubbish. I found him brusque and unkind. And I was frightened and worried. He wanted to give me antidepressants. I said I didn't want that. He sat down to write a prescription without further explanation. I asked for sleeping pills, but he refused. He prescribed vitamin B and something else he didn't explain, then he left. I felt that I'm not welcome in the healthcare system. I used to think I should wear a little tinkle bell like those infected with the plague long ago in the past. I could jingle the bell to give them all a chance to run away, all of them.'

For several women it was hard to clearly articulate their expectations of the consultation, except by saying 'I want to get help' or 'to get well'. In contrast, experiences of distress included all aspects of the encounter, including history-taking, the examination, the communication and the contact with the physician. The following unspoken, and unfulfilled, expectations of a 'creditable consultation' indirectly emerged as the women told what they had not received: to be taken seriously, to undergo a thorough physical examination, to have the time for an informative dialogue and to obtain an ongoing relationship with the physician.

Working hard to be taken seriously

What did the women do in their efforts to 'deserve' medical attention? The women we spoke to described different strategies to catch the physician's attention. In their efforts to be taken seriously, heard, seen and examined, they presented preferable bodily symptoms – manifestations that would be acceptable for the physician and for themselves:

> 'I didn't give any details about my private life. Well, I guess I had talked about my bad relationship and so on. I don't suppose you say straight out that you need help. You want it to be something physical.'

Although no pathology could be identified, the women maintained their bodily explanations. Ellinor continued: 'I was willing to be cut into pieces to figure out what was wrong with me.'

To get access to information, investigations, or therapeutic measures, the women disguised their demands in various ways. They referred to other authorities, 'I heard on TV' or 'My neighbor, who is a physician, said . . .', instead of speaking in terms of demands and wishes. Another way to cover up straightforward intentions was by flattering or appealing to the physician's supremacy, and presenting themselves as ignorant: 'So I called and said: "I don't understand anything." I made myself seem very stupid.' To plead, cry and to beg were described as extreme ways to gain attention, often with success.

> 'When I was really ill I was down on my knees for help. I have been crying my way through the medical service. If I hadn't . . . no one would have taken care of me . . . It was thanks to my continual asking.'

Being rejected was associated with strong feelings of distress. In order to maintain self-respect, the patients searched for alternative interpretations of their own and the physician's behavior. One way to accept the absence of a creditable diagnosis was to adopt a self-image of being incomprehensible, by mystifying the symptoms. 'Nothing works on me. I don't make sense to anybody, because I don't follow any medical laws.' Symptoms were given metaphysical explanations. For Sofie, the aching limbs were ruled by heavenly, meteorological or metallic laws:

> 'When the snow came, my fingers turned stiff and hard to bend.'

Although many of these women described constant pain and pilgrimages for help to different physicians, they also conveyed the image of the silent sufferer, never complaining, working beyond their power:

> 'For a long time I've thought, it will pass. I'm not the kind who worries much about myself; not until it's too late.'

Among the women, we frequently heard about a forgiving attitude toward their physicians. However, it easily turned into condemnation. After fruitless encounters, many patients expressed doubts about the physicians' knowledge, interest, and authority. Karen, who herself worked as a nurse at hospital, said:

> 'Well, to be honest. I think that many doctors are terribly ignorant. They know a lot of other things, but the back is just so complicated. There is probably a vast lack of knowledge.'

The ultimate position in the search for medical attention was 'to be under a doctor'. Delegating the responsibility to the physician might hold certain advantages. It implied shelter under a physician, whose task was to 'keep hold of her', her body and her recovery. On the other hand it held them back from taking active part in their own recoveries. How can we understand the grounds and the context for these patients' experiences of distrust, their strategies in the consultation and their search to be 'under a physician'? Let us have a look at the physicians' reactions.

Physicians have feelings, too

Physicians also have feelings and thoughts that have to be considered. Recognizing and reflecting on our own reactions might help us to master and restrain from damaging counter-transference (Hamberg and Johansson, 1999). Furthermore, self-reflection can be a pathway to personal development and may help a strained physician to understand his or her own tiredness, anger and feelings of helplessness. In this way, reflection may provide prevention against burnout symptoms.

Insoluble medical or non-medical problems, communication problems and personal issues from the physician's own life can cause negative feelings during difficult consultations. A point of departure in our research was our own frustration in not being able to help women with long-term pain. In several of the interview passages, we heard about contradictions and conflicts, and we experienced negative feelings ourselves.

Ella was 45 years old, divorced, with two children in their upper teens. She was a cleaner but had been sick-listed for several months due to myofascial pain. She had attended different rehabilitation programs without positive effect on her pain and had tried, and quit, several alternative jobs, saying they were too heavy. Ella described her previous situation at home:

> 'There is never any spare time. I never had any. I can never just sit and relax and do nothing. I always have to have something to do. I do some needlework, or I bake. There's always plenty of cake and buns at my place.'

We reacted strongly, became confused and a bit suspicious. As physicians, we had thoughts like, 'If she can achieve that much in the household, she ought to manage to work at least part-time in a paid job. Doesn't she want to work?,' Ella's description of her capabilities put the legitimacy of her sick certification in question and we became afraid of being deluded and misled.

At the same time, as women, we were also provoked. We compared her description with our own time left for cooking and sewing. Furthermore, our attitude was that 'womanliness is not grounded in housework' and in some respect, we felt accused by her prudence over housework. We perceived her description as an invitation to become intimate with the women's world. However, we rejected this invitation. Her world was not our world, her values were different from ours.

Ella was certainly aware of our doubts of the legitimacy of her symptoms, and she tried to convince us that she was the kind of person who really tries hard and does all that she can to get healthy and return to work. To support this stance, she had described her activity at home but rather than convince us of her sincerity, it increased our suspicions that she was being manipulative. Reactions such as these by the physician can make the patient a target of irritation and rejection, unless we become aware of them and find a way to clarify our questions and qualms.

Another example is a quotation from Janet, a 32-year-old home assistant with pre-school children. She suffered from back pain. At the time of this interview she worked full-time after a long period of sick-listing, but now she said:

> 'Well, I do manage the job but I'm totally exhausted when I come home. I'm always in a bad temper, nagging at the kids . . . simply cannot clean the dishes. I'm just too tired. I can't stand it like this. I need to be sick-listed.'

As physicians we felt embarrassed and had a feeling of failure: 'Is it really necessary that she be sick-listed again? It was such a step forward when she returned to work. It is not legal to certificate sick-listing due to heavy burdens at home . . . and the x-ray and all other tests were perfectly normal.' However, as mothers we could identify with her tiredness. This made it hard for us to comply with the official policy on sick-listing. We experienced a strong wish to find a solution that would work for this woman.

Although the position of physician implied doubts and suspicions against Janet, her position was strengthened because as a woman and mother the interviewer became an ally. There were many situations where it became obvious that motherhood and problems related to 'being a mother' were creating preconditions for feelings of solidarity and identification.

'As you know, the children come first!'

Concern and reflection

The patient-centered clinical method requires that the physician attend to feelings, emotions and moods as well as categorizing the illness. A positive attitude and an interest in the patient is more or less a precondition for a 'good consultation', and empathy for a patient usually facilitates patient-centeredness. Of course, we found many passages where our feelings were positive and empathetic, where we listened with interest, felt moved and sometimes upset and embarrassed on behalf of the women:

'My finances are bad. I have to plan everything. I have been in debt since we were married and I just have to prioritize . . . Only the necessary expenditures, the rent, the food and clothes for the kids. The rest has to wait. It is really bad, that you, . . . that you can't afford to be sick-listed although you need it. I can't afford being ill.'

In this situation, we experienced feelings of concern and affirmation. We saw the woman as a courageous fighter in an unfair economic system. She fit into the image of a brave, ambitious and suffering patient – a patient worthy of help. In follow-up questions, the interviewer acknowledged that it was a problematic situation. Our concern and emotional participation in this and similar interviews probably facilitated the women's narratives and as physicians, we felt more satisfied the more we got to know, the more we understood. This was a desired interaction, the physician acting supportive and according to a patient-centered approach.

However, strong positive feelings towards a patient might also blind the physician and sometimes hinder the patient's perspective from permeating the consultation. When a patient describes a situation the physician recognizes from his or her own life, there is a risk of identification that might lead the physician to stop being curious and to stop listening. The physician is convinced that she/he understands already.

'He was very nice and friendly . . . but he did not ask that much. His wife is also a secretary. He probably thought he knew what my back pain was all about.'

If the patient believes that a certain experience, question or demand might alter the physician's benevolent attitude, she might choose to veil her wishes. It is common that patients avoid complaining about ineffective drugs and treatments. They don't want to make the physician disappointed and risk the loss of the advantageous relationship.

'I know that you want me to go to the physiotherapist and that you think it's good . . . but if you only knew what I feel inside.'

The examples illustrate how similarities and differences between patients and their physicians in the areas of attitudes, habits and values constitute important features of the patient–physician relationship. Reflecting on such aspects of communication is an important part of a patient-centered approach. Furthermore, as illustrated above, like all human beings, physicians might react in different ways depending on what aspect of personality and what ideas are triggered in a certain situation. Nevertheless, the physicians' own feelings in consultations are, as yet, neglected areas in clinical practice as well as research.

We have reflected further on the attitudes we felt towards the women as physicians, women and mothers. In other situations it might be rewarding to reflect on consultations from other viewpoints. Some example are: values about healthy eating and weight reduction in a situation where the patient prefers eating fast and fat food on the street corner and the physician wants her to slim; or values and ideas about smoking, when the patient who has stopped smoking sees a physician who smells of tobacco.

Of course, readers might not react like we did to the quotations. As physicians, we differ not only according to gender, ethnicity, age and cultural background; we also have different interests, political preferences and values which have an impact on our reactions and decisions. Hitherto we have focused on the patient's and the physician's reactions and feelings. Let us now integrate the discussion and scrutinize the consultation, the context in which these reactions are taking place.

The biomedical discourse of the consultation context

From the women's narratives, reinforced by the physician's reactions, we find it striking how biological considerations may push the diagnostic procedures, and dominate the patient–physician interaction. The physician's task is to help the patient by investigating, finding a diagnosis and giving adequate treatment. The physician, therefore, must always have his or her eyes and ears open for signs and signals of diseases, and be prepared to try to find out what could improve the health of each single patient.

The women in our study tried to emphasize their bodily symptoms as a way to get what they needed. They did not want the pain to be classified as something psychological. By describing the pain in intense and dramatic ways, presenting the suffering as hard and sometimes unbearable and demanding somatic investigations, the patients put a heavy responsibility on the physicians to help. Patients with medically unexplained problems are sometimes labeled 'somatizers'. However, it might be that it is the physicians who induce or contribute to somatization (Campion *et al.*, 1992). When patients present psychosocial aspects, it is common that physicians lose interest. They interrupt, do not comment or change the theme of discussion and, in doing so, signal what is of importance and what is not (Salmon and May, 1995). Often, the physician wants to exclude somatic disorders first and then, if 'nothing' is found, there is a risk that the patient's symptoms are reduced to pure psychology (Bazanger, 1993).

To characterize a patient as 'somatizing' or a 'somatizer' means to classify her as deviant in behavior, and thereby unaware of connections between psychological circumstances and bodily sensations. Although somatization is seldom mentioned as a diagnosis in primary care, the model of somatization delineates psychodynamic as well as cognitive models for treatment and rehabilitation of patients with CMP. This creates problems. For patients with long-term pain the recommendation of treatment focused on behavior holds a potential for stigmatization. The patients feel that their pain is being questioned and that they are responsible for and guilty over the pain. As a result, the patient tries to defend herself, escape the feelings of guilt and instead reveal the physician as incompetent. A struggle for respect, power and preferential right of interpretation starts.

Power asymmetry in the patient–physician relationship

In Western culture, the physician's role is still characterized by high status, power and control. Ethical, administrative and legislative guidelines regulate what is right and legal to do as a physician. These are ethical commitments – to do good and be the patient's humble servant – but at the same time, the physician faces political demands for time-effective care and requests to lower healthcare costs. Here, physician and patient may have different expectations and interests (Bendelow and Williams, 1996). Still, in the encounter the traditional notion is that the physician is leading and the patient is following, counteracting a patient-centered approach. The women in our study also admitted that they felt the physician's positional power to be obstructive. Lena said:

> 'I've always been afraid of physicians. I place them that high, and I am down here. Frankly, I am a little bit afraid of you too. I've been thinking . . . after all . . . why should I expose myself to . . . a complete stranger?'

The women described situations where their attempts to question and discuss assumptions were met by demeaning, paternalistic comments such as 'That was pure rubbish' or 'You see, now it is this way . . .'. Physicians find it problematic to handle distrust and to demonstrate their own uncertainty. The physicians' attitudes described by the patients in the study, such as ignoring, disregarding and rejecting, can also be interpreted as the physicians' ways to master feelings of being threatened or failing. These attitudes are important to identify, as they cause misunderstanding, distrust and dissatisfaction which may intensify health utilization and 'doctor-shopping'.

An immediate reaction from the physician towards a demanding patient might be fighting back and defending the physician's privilege to make decisions about diagnosis and treatment. It is more beneficial for the patient–physician relationship if we realize our frustrated feelings as signals and warnings. It would be better to hesitate, reflect and try to find questions that can open up discussion. There might be important information or messages from the patient that are missed or overlooked. Moreover, we have to be aware of strong, positive feelings, too, because they also result in the patient's voice being silenced.

> 'You were so supportive, eager to help and convinced that it was something pressing on my nerves in the shoulder . . . you did not listen when I tried to say it had to be something else. I gave up . . .'

The impact of gender

Another issue embedded in the context of the patient–clinician relationship is gender, i.e. the biological sex as well as the socially constructed identity of 'womanliness' and 'manliness' (West, 1993). The impact of gender on the consultation is not just something that happens, but it can also serve particular purposes for the individuals taking part. During our research project, when we scrutinized the patient–physician interaction, we uncovered how gender stereotypes present themselves. When the women talked about 'the physician', they described 'him' as a male stereotype; strong, decisive, but also brusque and rejecting. Their ambiguous expectations about women physicians were also evident. The women expected a female physician to be caring, accommodating and understanding, but a male physician to be authoritarian and decisive. As Alice pondered about physicians and gender:

'I think a female doctor really would listen and care about my problems . . . but . . . would she prescribe Valium, if I asked, as my current doctor does?'

Men and women patients differ in the way they elaborate their complaints, i.e. they differ in illness behavior. Women report more symptoms, both physical and mental, and utilize the health service more extensively than men do. When presenting their symptoms, women refer more to other people, such as family, friends and colleagues, than men do, and they more often express emotional troubles related to sex roles (Borges and Waitzkin, 1995). Women patients can take advantage of a socially ascribed, feminine help-seeking behavior, i.e. to report and discuss feelings and discomfort, and to involve healthcare. Physicians, on the other hand, might take advantage, such as goodwill, status and compliance, and not invite women patients into the sick role.

The physician's gender seems to be of little importance when it concerns the medical management of patients' health problems (Sayer and Britt, 1996). However, men and women physicians perform differently in the verbal part of the consultation as well as in non-verbal communication (West, 1993). Men physicians behave in a more imposing and presumptuous manner, females in a more attentive and non-directive manner. In a Dutch study, female family physicians had longer consultations. This was partly explained by the fact that more health problems were presented to female physicians compared to their male colleagues (Van den Brink-Muinen *et al.*, 1994). In England, women physicians displayed a more patient-centered style, asked more open questions and offered greater attention to their patients (Law and Britten, 1996).

Yet, we want to warn against a tendency to promote sex-stereotyped theories about physicians' behavior when we talk about women and men as separate groups and homogenous entities. All women are not attentive towards their patients and all men don't react in the same way. In our study, it became evident that women physicians might have difficulties in consultations with women patients due to gender-related demands (Hamberg and Johansson, 1999). Both similarities and differences between men and women are situational and interactional. Patients' expectations shape physicians' conduct as well. If a woman physician is considered to be more empathetic than a man, she might act and behave accordingly, while it might be hard for a man to contradict the presumed 'maleness' in the status of a physician, connected to status-determining tracks such as high wages, authority, expertise and power.

However, being aware of the gendered patient–physician relationship can be a strength, helping us navigate through the limitations and develop other possibilities. The physician who maintains that medicine is gender-neutral will not be able to decipher his or her role as a participant in the gendered processes where clinical knowledge is produced and shared. Realizing the significance of gender, the physician may become a more qualified and attentive reader of medical signs, as well as difficult consultations.

Judith Smith has great respect for Dr Jamesson. She knows he is a busy man and she tries to be accurate when she sees him, as she is afraid he will see her as a hypochondriac crock. At the same time, she depends on his empathy and understanding. Consequently, Judith spends a lot of time thinking about how she is going to present her complaints in a way that will be taken seriously. She does not want him to believe that she is lazy or reluctant to work, because she loves to be at work and is proud to fulfill her duties.

The last time Judith visited Dr Jamesson she asked for a referral to a specialist in rheumatology. He examined her joints and tense muscles carefully, and said there were no signs of rheumatism. Later, they spent some time discussing her thoughts and ideas about the cause of her pain. She then told him about her friend who died from breast cancer after several years of rheumatoid arthritis. Although he did not approve her wish for a referral he was still concerned, examined her breasts and arranged to send her for a mammogram. She felt that she could trust him when he said that further investigations were not indicated. When he asked her why she did not show up for the physiotherapist appointment, he did not even seem to be criticizing her. He rather sounded curious, and she told him about her mother-in-law, who had almost set the house on fire last week. He said that he should visit Greg's mother and try to see if he could do anything to help – it might even be possible to get room for her at the nursing home.

Dr Jamesson felt a bit ashamed that he did not know that old Mrs Smith was so much worse with her Alzheimer's symptoms. He could remember that Judith had mentioned it in passing some time ago, but then he did not grasp the severity of the problem. He thought, 'It must be a time-consuming burden to care for the old lady . . . How does Judith piece her time together?' Nevertheless, on the whole, Dr Jamesson was satisfied with the outcome of this consultation. Something had happened in his relationship with Judith. She had not repeated the same story, but rather revealed that she was afraid of a serious disease. If he could not help her with anything else, he could at least deal with her fear of cancer.

Empowering the patient by reframing the discourse

Kirsti Malterud

After several years of clinical practice, I found myself repeatedly stuck with patients presenting medically unexplained problems. They came to me with long-lasting, painful and vague conditions where no objective findings could be demonstrated (Malterud, 1987). A considerable proportion of these patients suffered from CMP syndromes, and most of them were women. Evidence told me that these problems comprised a considerable proportion of women's health problems in general. Medical textbooks offered no solutions for understanding and management except various psychiatric diagnoses, which most often were rejected by the patients. Feelings of helplessness provoked my professional identity of being in charge, and were sometimes, unfortunately, transformed into more aggressive behavior, where I shamefully realized that my disapproving attitudes had been blamed on the patient. Below, I will share some of my strategies and experiences of trying to reframe the discourse in a systematic way. I wanted to expand the understanding of the patient's agenda, trusting the patient's resources.

When something I said made a difference

The obvious suffering of the patients told me that the resolution was not to deny or discard their illness. Gradually, the 'unexplained' problems became more available for understanding and management. Experience gently taught me the art of recognizing patterns of symptom presentation, comparing these to the individual's particular needs and resources and subsequently transferring this understanding into medical management, which sometimes seemed to work. Over the years, I acquired various clinical strategies and a feeling of being more skillful replaced my helplessness. My enthusiasm was triggered by events where something I said somehow seemed to make a major difference, not just regarding emotions, but even more on a problem-solving level. I felt that such incidents concerned shared knowledge, perhaps made available by empowering the voice of the woman by means of something I did or said; a key to mutual understanding that served to unlock previously closed gateways (Malterud, 1992, 1999, 2000).

Communication is a strong agent for gendered interaction, and the consultation may reproduce sociocultural patterns of power, leaving limited voice for the patient who is in a subordinate position (Borges and Waitzkin, 1995). Empowerment means to redistribute power and strengthen the underprivileged. According to critical theory, empowerment for personal and political liberation can be promoted by communicative action. I decided to elaborate my communication style to expand the empowered space for the patient in a more conscious way, by turning intuitive talk into a clinical method.

I had occasionally experienced that my tacit clinical knowledge included certain communicative skills, including questions that gave access to further understanding. These skills were accomplished intuitively and casually, and I was not able to account for what I said or how it worked. Realizing that my ways of asking might lead to major differences as a key to unlocking my understanding of the woman's problem, I became inspired to identify and refine specific components of my communicative style as an action-research project in my own practice, based on qualitative material from audiotaped consultations and field-notes (Malterud, 1999).

I decided to systematize my best experiences by developing a communicative method intended to empower the voices of women patients suffering from medically unexplained problems. My hypothesis was that empowerment would promote exchange of medically relevant information. My approach was to develop simple communicative clues 'key questions' intended to invite the patient to share her knowledge. The key questions, all four of them, were designed as speech acts, conversational elements that hold a potential to promote action (Austin, 1982).

Exploring the patient's agenda by means of key questions

The key questions were designed to elucidate different aspects of the patient's agenda. I wanted to invite her to share with me her knowledge about problem definition, causal beliefs, expected actions from the physician and previous experiences of management. Problem definition and expected actions from the physicians are related to the concept of 'patient's expectations' in the patient-centered clinical method, causal beliefs are related to 'patient's ideas', while knowledge about previous experiences of management can be essential for 'finding common ground'. However, the key questions presented here explore more specifically different aspects of the patient's agenda. The four questions were not meant to be used in the same consultation, but designed as tools for the deliberate pursuit of different perspectives that might be of different significance in different consultations.

Through an elaborate development process, I arrived at the following key questions:

Problem definition:
'What would you, really most of all, want me to do for you today?'

Causal beliefs:
'What do you yourself think is the reason for x?' (x means the health complaint described in the woman's own words)

when necessary, complemented with:

'Yes, we'll certainly find out about that – but I am sure you have been thinking of what might be the causes of x.'

and, when necessary, even complemented with:

'Since you have suffered from x for y days – you must have been thinking of its possible causes.'

Expected actions from the physician:
'What do you think I should do with x – I'm sure you have thought of that before you came here?'

Previous experiences of management
'What have you so far found to be the best way of managing the illness?'

Make your own key questions, while keeping some issues in mind

You should not consider these questions as magic formulas, directly transferable word by word, but rather as examples and points of departure for your own wording. The skillful and flexible clinician may develop his or her own key questions, hopefully inspired by the intentions, examples and empowering potentials of these phrasings, yet anchored in his or her own personal language. Through pragmatic linguistic analysis I identified the potentially empowering strength of these key questions as related to:

- open-ended questions, implying the existence of multiple response alternatives beyond the imagination of the doctor
- terms implying concrete connections to reality, anchoring the conversation to the actual encounter
- invitation to the woman's potentials of imagination, reminding her of her problem-solving resources

- stating the role of the patient as a source of knowledge by acknowledging her experiences
- repetitively sanctioning the patient's medical language, verifying the competence claimed by her own words
- humourous invitation to mutuality, to avoid embarrassing the woman delivering her own version of the situation
- an option of dignified retreat, signalling that the patient is in charge of defining her own position
- claiming the doctor's readiness for responsibility, proving that problem solving is going to be a matter of co-operation.

The patient's answers to the key questions expanded my understanding of her agenda. I obtained access to information concerning life conditions in the patients, assumed to affect the origins and dynamics of their health complaints, the resulting presentation of symptoms and their perceived needs of health services. The first issue has already been dealt with in Chapter 3. Here, I shall therefore prioritize the latter ones, on symptom presentation and perceived needs.

How is the patient's symptom presentation influenced by context?

The presentation of health complaints in the encounter between patient and physician is influenced by standards of sick-role behavior. We may expect a woman patient to claim responsibility for the emotional climate of the patient–physician relationship – even on the premises of the doctor. The analysis of the material focused on how the symptom presentation may be shaped by the patient's need to convey to the healthcare provider a proper image of herself.

When patients suffer from slight anxiety, and do not really believe their symptoms are due to serious disease, the conversation may become very complex. To avoid the labelling of hypochondriasis, they may present their fears in a vague way. When women believe their health complaints to be their own fault, they also may conceal their health beliefs, hoping not to be blamed for being sick. Such thoughts may occur independently of who is actually to blame for the real causality and origins of the symptoms.

Women suffering from an overload of demands and expectations may present their resulting health complaints by trying to evade the physician's unrealistic recommendations to reduce stress and strain. A shameful feeling of how they should have prevented the health complaints can be hidden behind a laborious and overdetailed presentation of the symptoms, with a resulting misunderstanding in the doctor. In contrast, when given the possibility of presenting their own understanding of causality and dynamics of the health complaint, women patients may give very precise and well-defined descriptions of their complaints.

What does the patient expect?

When asked the key question on expected actions from the physician, the patients mentioned a variety of actions they hoped the doctor would provide. The great diversity reminds us of the significance of an individualized approach, checking out with the patient about how specific desires and needs may be situated (Malterud, 2000). To inspire the reader, some examples are presented.

Specific wishes or just support?

Some of the women were not able to express their expectations in more detail. However, by answering the key question, they nevertheless made it perfectly clear that they came to the doctor with very particular requests that usually dealt with a wish to know more:

> The patient (aged 65) had been tired for a while and previously her creatinine level had been elevated. At the next test, her values were normal. She came back to discuss what to do. Her answer to the key question was: 'I leave it completely to the doctor – I don't even think of it. I just needed to have an answer.'

The patient does not always anticipate further investigation or treatment even though her symptoms may be bothering her. Sometimes, she wants the physician to support her belief that she will not suffer any loss or danger by just awaiting the situation. This is a way to escape the responsibility that something specific should have been done.

> Four weeks prior to her visit to the doctor, a woman of 59 hit her head on a luggage rack on the train. When she returned back home, she went to her physician who told her that she had a minor concussion. She recovered steadily, but still felt dizzy and had a headache in stressed situations. She answered my question like this:
>
> > 'I just wanted to know whether you usually feel like this in such situations. Because my friend's daughter experienced something similar,

I guess nearly two years ago. She just turned 37. And she was told to lie down, but I guess she did not follow the advice as strictly as she should. So she went on a disability pension due to this. I was afraid that if I did not take this sufficiently seriously, I might also keep my symptoms and not be able to do anything at all.'

There were no neurological findings, and she was clearly feeling better. Her friends thought she needed an x-ray, but she was prepared to wait unless that would be risky for her.

A proper examination

A symptom can produce a very specific perception in the patient of what is wrong with her. She may have considered what is needed to confirm or discard this conception – often very simple actions with a potential for providing safety, so long as the physician knows what her thinking is on this matter.

A woman of 65 had previously consulted me several times for her backache. The x-rays demonstrated degenerative signs of ageing. She visited because the pain had become worse the last week. Her answer was this:

'I thought that maybe you would examine my back. If perhaps you found a lump or something. It feels as if I had a knife in my back which was pulled out. Yes – just find out whether there is something abnormal – I can't reach around there, so I won't be able to find out myself.'

No lump could be found, but her muscles were very tense and painful at the left upper lumbar area where the 'knife' had been felt.

The patient may have very specific ideas about what could be done to provide an explanation of her symptoms. This does not necessarily mean that she expects a referral, although she may have anticipated this possibility.

A 62-year-old woman was previously healthy, until she a few days earlier fell against the frame of a door and hit her back. She showed signs of pain, but did not seem to be especially worried. Her answer to the key question was this:

'You know, my only concern is to have a proper examination. It feels like something pressing. And then, if you find an x-ray to be necessary, well – if I should admit that I thought of anything at all, that is what came to my thoughts.'

She was relieved when I concluded after the clinical exam that I did not think she would need a referral. A week later she called and said she was fully recovered and doing her usual things.

Acknowledging previous experiences and present needs

Previous treatment experiences provide significant contributions to the shaping of the patient's expectations of what should be done. If the patient previously had gone through actions that gave her little benefit, she would not be happy to repeat the same procedure. Effective approaches may be more tempting, even when the actual problem is other than what the treatment was intended for.

> A 66-year-old woman had for years been suffering from a painful hip and periods of pain in her left shoulder. An appointment was made to discuss her shoulder pain, but during the visit, the hip was identified as even more troublesome. She answered the key question:
>
> > 'As for my hip – I had treatments like heat and massage. That is many years ago, but it kept me well for a long time. That might perhaps help me? You would know; I was here previously with my shoulder. I was told that I should go home, lift my iron and move it all around. But I did that, and still I am not able to lift the arm as I would like to. And it is painful when I stretch to put on my bra. So I don't know what to do with this arm; I really don't know. No, if I am going to have treatment, I will need massage. No electric devices.'
>
> It would have been senseless to suggest that this woman should go home and do exercises for her shoulder. It was useful for me to hear about her reluctance regarding ultrasound and electrotherapy, which might have activated her uneasiness toward any kind of physiotherapy. I referred her for heat, massage and selected exercises.

Women often listen to others and share responsibility for other people's problems and worries. At the same time, they hope that someone will listen to their worries when they are in need. If they experience a lack of space for them and their problems, they may feel abandoned. Perhaps the woman's most important expectation is that her physician will give her the space she needs (Malterud, 2000).

> A woman of 45 started by briefly describing her considerable family problems, and told me that recently she had felt dizzy and tired. She had

previously seen another physician for these matters, but felt that she had not been helped. Her presentation demonstrated a clear insight into the connections between her symptoms and her life situation. I thought that maybe she still wanted a physical investigation. However, her answer to the key question was:

'You know, I was wondering quite a lot; somehow, I don't know what to do, because it makes no sense to speak to the physician I saw before. He sat there, writing at his computer. He didn't talk to me at all, writing while I talked, so I kept wondering whether it was about what I said, or about other patients he had just seen an hour ago or something. It was very frustrating. At my last visit, I felt he urged me out of his office, he put on his shoes and seemed to be on his way home. There were still a lot of people in the waiting room, no system in the line or something, and a woman asked to come before me, because she was supposed to have her appointment an hour earlier. So I felt frustrated and decided that I could not continue seeing that doctor. He gives me no understanding. I just needed someone who would listen to me.'

We talked for 15 minutes, and I did not say much. She had her husband join her for the family counselor, and later returned to me for other problems.

Knowing that the doctor cannot solve the problem

Sometimes, the patient knows well that the physician cannot solve her problems. Still, she attends for a visit. This might mislead the provider into believing that the woman does not trust her own coping abilities. Perhaps she needs to use the physician as one to whom she can declare her own strength.

I saw a 51-year-old woman who was on long-term sick leave after a period of burn-out at work. She loved her demanding job, although it had taken energy beyond the capacity of her body. Her feelings of responsibility towards her work were intense, and it was not easy for her to refuse tasks where resources were too small for appropriate accomplishment. She responded:

'I guess I am the one who needs to do something to stop this rat race, although this is not easy, considering all these people to whom we are accountable.'

My role during her sick leave was to support her in developing a strategy where she gradually learned how far she wanted to stretch herself, elaborating methods for setting limits when needed.

Approaching the patient's strength and resources

Communicative empowerment implies more than understanding disease and risk factors. The attitudes of contemporary medicine, labeled as the risk epidemic, may contribute to blaming the victims of disease, neglecting individual and collective strength (Skolbekken, 1995). The sociologist Antonovsky challenged this view of health and disease by introducing the concept of *salutogenesis* (genesis = origin, saluto = health), looking for resources that keep people healthy (Antonovsky, 1979). Behavioral and psychoimmunoneurological medical research substantiates the potential for human self-healing and its relationship to the internal and external context of the individual. In the process of chronic disease, such as CMP, salutogenic perspectives are important remedies for empowerment, acknowledgment and hope in the pursuit of a revised notion of being healthy, even in a life of pain.

The family physician is in the privileged position of being able to observe the power of the human body's capacity for repair and restoration. The patient-centered clinical method highlights the voice of the patient as a valid source of medical knowledge. Hollnagel and Malterud have presented 'The health resource/risk balance' model, a salutogenic and patient-centered consultation model that shifts the attention of the physician from objective risk factors in patients to their self-assessed personal health resources (Hollnagel and Malterud, 1995). This model, elaborated from the original patient-centered clinical method, encourages the doctor to identify and combine the agendas of pathogenesis and risk factors with salutogenesis and health resources, as well as the agendas of doctor-assessment with patient-assessment.

According to Antonovsky, general resistance resources, such as social class and network, facilitate health in most people. Hollnagel and Malterud introduce the concept of *self-assessed personal health resources*, denoting the individual's subjective experience and perception of qualities or strategies which she/he thinks maintain her/his health, irrespective of empirical evidence about health effects (Hollnagel and Malterud, 1995). Self-assessed health resources can only be obtained through an individualized approach, such as the patient-centered clinical method. Shared understanding of the health resources observed by the physician and the patients' self-assessed health resources is the basis of patient-centered salutogenesis in clinical practice.

Self-assessed health resources in women patients

The theoretical framework presented above was the starting point for a study we did in our own practices. The study included development and implementation of a key question on self-assessed health resources (Malterud and Hollnagel, 1997, 1998). To inspire the reader to look for resources in patients with CMP, I shall present some of the answers from 37 women, who were posed the following resource key question:

'We cannot talk only about problems. I also want to hear about your strong sides. Which of these strong sides do you normally use to stay (or become) well?'

The women spoke about health resources related to internal strength mobilized by external strain, interactive networks within and outside the family, lifestyle practices, physical and social activity, acceptance and facilitation of the natural course of disease and constitution.

Mastering the art of strain and indispensability

The key question responses showed that internal strength makes it possible for the women to cope with tasks and expectations which just have to be met, although some of them remarked that it might be almost too much for them. The women spoke about personal potentials such as stubbornness and endurance, internal demands to keep going, forcing themselves, and experiences which support the conviction that the task is essential and therefore must be fulfilled:

'In my life I have been in lots of strained situations, and I know that I shall manage it in one way or the other. I am sure I shall cope with this one as well. I believe this is what keeps me going.'

External demands related to the women's caring role in the family (and sometimes at work) create the frame from which health resources may be mobilized. Activities of daily life have to be performed and there is no room for sickness. The women experienced themselves as indispensable, in a way which paradoxically provided the strength to keep going. This seemed to be especially important when the demands were related to needs of the children. Some of the women described these aspects as stressful and unpleasant, while others perceived the responsibilities of caring as positive experiences which counteracted illness:

'It is a good alternative to be with the children instead of sinking down into depression.'

Some reported how they suppressed their emotions, in order to control the situation; not to be a burden to anyone else, and to prevent others from being bothered:

'Mostly, I keep quiet and don't tell anybody. But it may also depend on the kind of problem, whether I can talk to somebody about it.'

Living a healthy life among other people

A common theme was the positive experience of interacting with other people, adults or children. Human interactions at home or at work seemed to produce strength and growth, promote activity and joy and prevent loneliness:

'Being together with my children helps me get up and out.'

The women said that prior experiences of talking about their problems had contributed to solutions. Discussing sharing of household responsibilities or finding joint solutions to common problems with their husbands were mentioned as potentials for change. Sharing problems with family members, friends or professionals had led to caring support and had prevented development of symptoms and depression:

'I used to talk to other people, especially my boyfriend.'

Traditional lifestyle elements were mentioned by several patients. Many spoke about dietary habits which are known to promote a healthy life, such as salad, vegetables, brown bread, fish and curdled milk. Some described their menu in great detail, or emphasized the regularity or variety of their meals. Resisted temptations were also mentioned, and many women said they were dieting to control their weight. Some used vitamins, cod-liver oil or calcium tablets:

'My eating habits are quite healthy. We eat a lot of salad and vegetables and normally we use brown bread.'

A lot of the women took regular physical exercise to keep fit; many went walking, some even for hours every day, in the woods or in the neighborhood. Other fitness activities such as cycling, running or aerobics were very common, though often described as a duty which must be accomplished, or as something which they failed to achieve. The women frequently used phrases like 'clever' or 'not so clever' about themselves. But the joy of being in bodily activity was nevertheless a substantial part:

> 'I enjoy my walks in the woods and the fields. I am interested in outdoor activities and I love to do these kinds of things.'

Activities may prevent symptoms

For several women, being active was given as one of their health resources. Being ill meant feeling useless, while lying in bed was dull and produced a negative feeling. The activities were not related to fitness exercises, but to ordinary, daily-life events. One woman with a psychiatric disease had found, during her hospital stay, that physical activity might prevent a relapse of symptoms.

> 'I like to be active. Due to this, I feel a bit useless now that I am at home, because I am not able to do so much. I start with things which I am not able to finish. But being active, and especially outdoors feels good to me.'

Activities at home and in the family were often reported as health resources. Also, women described housework, cooking, cleaning, gardening or care-taking as a resource:

> 'Sometimes I go for walks. And then do the housework. If we are having guests, I make the food. Several times a week I take care of my grandchild. I meet her at school and that sort of thing.'

For some women, activities were a means of letting off steam, e.g. cycling, swimming or manual household activities. This contrasted with their regular paid work. Some of them spoke about such activities as a way of escaping the stress of daily life or nagging symptoms like migraine:

> 'The pain – I cannot move away from it. But it is most prominent when I lie in bed. By just doing something, I try to get rid of it, although the migraine will not just leave me completely.'

Self-care

It was a common experience that many problems resolved with time. The women apparently knew something about the natural course of disease and about behavior which promoted a positive outcome. They told us that believing things would take their own course made them relax, assuming that nothing special had to be done:

'I always just wait, hoping that it will soon be over.'

A few women mentioned strategies from which they actively got rest or relief, e.g. a rest after dinner, staying in bed when they were ill, sleeping through influenza or listening to the signals from the body:

'When I am ill, I just go to bed, say, for three days. I have found that this is the most effective remedy. I have very good experiences with this approach. I get a week's sick leave from work and stay quiet. This has helped me.'

Some women spoke about taking care of themselves by means of pleasant leisure activities (going to the cinema, reading a book, having an enjoyable time at home) or by keeping a distance from stressful situations, e.g. by sailing, or ignoring the telephone:

'I watch a film or read a good book, when there is peace and quiet in the house.'

Constitutional components were also reported. Some women referred to their family as healthy, or a family with good genetic material. They also described personal characteristics which may enhance their health, such as good humor, optimism, joy of life, loyalty or strength:

'In our family we have an exceptionally high tolerance for pain. All my sisters and brothers are like that, and my mother as well.'

Empowerment in practice

The key-question experiences have taught us how feelings of professional helplessness can be replaced by shared understanding and collaboration. The findings propose that the medical discourse can be reframed towards more empowering approaches. Although the empowerment was intended to be directed towards the patients, I also found myself feeling empowered as a primary care physician by being able to understand more of what is going on.

The medical needs and expectations of patients seeking care are shaped by the nature of the problem, the medical competence of the clinician and by the options of change in favor of health in the life of the patient. The key-question strategy gave access to several strategies for resource, mobilizing strategies perceived as adequate by the patients themselves.

Some health complaints raise the needs of medical clarification more than expectation of cure. Although the doctor may expect the patient to crave treatment, his or her real requirements and needs could rather be about labeling and explanation of the illness. In some patients, the most important task of the clinician would be to confirm the patient's dignity in a strained life situation. The patient-centered clinical method assumes that care must be based upon the patient's own definition of her health disorder. This requires a high level of attentiveness in the physician. The relief of responsibility through medical care should be balanced by an active transfer of power to the patient. Recognizing and supporting the agency of the patient in his or her own life can be facilitated when the physician identifies and approves of the patient's strong points.

Patients with myofascial pain syndromes sometimes feel discarded by their physician. One explanation for this might be the perception of the healthcare provider as realizing that the complaints arise on the surface of extensive 'non-medical' sociocultural or structural problems, such as the layers of oppression described by Candib in the previous chapter. In such cases, it is especially important that primary care problem-solving is based on the patient's insight into his or her life situation, which may enable the physician to understand the dynamics of the symptoms. The patient may still not expect the physician to solve the basic problems, but nevertheless provide definite elements of problems that can be approached and perhaps even solved by the medical encounter. However, the family physician will need to be warned against an omnipotent attitude, which will lead to a feeling of helplessness in the healthcare provider as well as in the patient. By understanding where the patient is, the physician may be able to help.

Potentials, pitfalls and challenges for the physician

I shall close this chapter by summarizing some recommendations and warnings to support the relationship between patients with CMP and their physicians (Malterud, 2000).

Strategies in clinical practice

- Acknowledge the woman's suffering, even when you are not able to understand or explain it.
- Consider the situation as a challenge, not a threat: stay curious.

- Explore the woman's agenda, including the problem definition, thoughts about origins, expectations towards healthcare, experiences of management, and identify her strong points.
- Learn more about the relationships between living conditions and health (remember, especially, abuse and disempowerment).
- Don't rely on universal solutions: each patient is an individual who can be asked and trusted.

Specific warnings

- Stay away from simple psychosocial explanations: bodily complaints are not necessarily in people's minds.
- Comprehensive and purposeful somatic assessment is necessary and may need to be repeated.
- Stay away from endless diagnostic marathons: the answer is not always a diagnosis, although you and the patient will need to name the condition together.
- Respect privacy beyond what you need to know: patient-centeredness is not the same as intrusiveness, and intimate information requires trust.
- Don't just explain the conclusion to the patient: truth needs to be negotiated.
- Don't expect a cure: care may be sufficient, but don't forget that some actually may recover.

References

Antonovsky A (1979) *Health, Stress and Coping: new perspective on mental and physical well-being.* Jossey-Bass Publishers, Washington DC.

Austin JL (1982) *How to Do Things with Words* (2e). Oxford University Press, Oxford.

Bazanger I (1993) Deciphering chronic pain. *Sociol Health Illness.* **14**: 219–29.

Bendelow G and Williams S (1996) The end of the road?: lay views on a pain relief clinic. *Soc Sci Med.* **43**: 1127–36.

Borges S and Waitzkin H (1995) Women's narratives in primary care medical encounters. *Women Health.* **23**: 29–56.

Campion PD, Butler NM and Cox AD (1992) Principle agendas of doctors and patients in general practice. *Fam Pract.* **9**: 181–90.

Hahn SR, Kroenke K, Spitzer RL *et al.* (1996) The difficult patient: prevalence, psychopathology and functional impairment. *J Gen Intern Med.* **11**: 1–8.

Hamberg K and Johansson EE (1999) Practitioner, researcher and gender conflict in a qualitative study. *Qual Health Res.* **9**: 455–67.

Hollnagel H and Malterud K (1995) Shifting attention from objective risk factors to patients' self-assessed health resources: a clinical model for general practice. *Fam Pract.* **12**: 423–9.

Johansson EE, Hamberg K, Lindgren G and Westman G (1996) 'I've been crying my way': qualitative analysis of a group of female patients' consultation experiences. *Fam Pract.* **13**: 498–503.

Law SAT and Britten N (1996) Factors that influence the patient-centredness of a consultation. *Br J Gen Pract.* **45**: 520–4.

Malterud K (1987) Illness and disease in female patients: I. Pitfalls and inadequacies of primary healthcare classification systems: a theoretical review. *Scand J Prim Health Care.* **5**: 205–9.

Malterud K (1992) Women's 'undefined' disorders: a challenge for clinical communication. *Fam Pract.* **9**: 299–303.

Malterud K (1999) Making changes with key questions in medical practices: studying what makes a difference. In: BF Crabtree and WL Miller (eds) *Doing Qualitative Research* (2e). Sage Publications, Thousand Oaks, CA.

Malterud K (2000) Symptoms as a source of medical knowledge: understanding medically unexplained disorders in women. *Fam Med.* **32**: 417–25.

Malterud K and Hollnagel H (1997) Women's self-assessed personal health resources. *Scand J Prim Health Care.* **15**: 163–8.

Malterud K and Hollnagel H (1998) Talking with women about personal health resources in general practice: key questions about salutogenesis. *Scand J Prim Health Care.* **16**: 66–71.

Pendleton D, Schofield T, Tate P and Havelock P (1984) *The Consultation: an approach to learning and teaching.* Oxford Medical Publications, Oxford.

Salmon P and May CR (1995) Patients' influence on doctors' behavior: a case study of patient strategies in somatization. *Int J Psychiatry Med.* **25**: 319–29.

Sayer GP and Britt H (1996) Sex differences in morbidity: a case of discrimination in general practice. *Soc Sci Med.* **42**: 257–64.

Schwenk TL, Marquez JT, Lefever RD and Cohen M (1989) Physician and patient determinants of difficult physician–patient relationship. *J Fam Pract.* **28**: 59–63.

Skolbekken JA (1995) The risk epidemic in medical journals. *Soc Sci Med.* **40**: 291–305.

Van den Brink-Muinen A, de Bakker DH and Bensing JM (1994) Consultations for women's health problems: factors influencing women's choice of sex of general practitioner. *Br J Gen Pract.* **44**: 205–10.

West C (1993) Reconceptualizing gender in physician–patient relationship. *Soc Sci Med.* **36**: 57–66.

6

Management of chronic myofascial pain: finding common ground

After all these painful years, Judith Smith has gained a comprehensive experience from a broad variety of treament modalities. She is astonished to conclude that treatment seemingly in fashion eight years ago, such as resting, now seems to be completely abandoned. Dr Jamesson assures her that evidence is changing, but she does not understand why this is so. Knowledge is knowledge — or is it not? Judith Smith has been prescribed anti-inflammatory drugs as painkillers, but stopped this medication because her stomach was hurting. She has been offered brief therapy sessions, which helped her for a while. One physician even asked her to write notes about her ailments. Her physiotherapist gave her exercises to do and massage. She enjoyed the latter, and still tries to maintain the former. After some periods of sick-listing, the hospital enrolled her in a rehabilitation group for employees with various problems. In the beginning, she was a bit reluctant, because the other participants were younger and seemed more able-bodied than herself. However, when she got to know them, she experienced recognition as well as support from them. Sometimes, she misses the period when she went to the group. Her sister-in-law suggested that she should see an acupuncturist, and the treatment somehow seems to relieve her pain. However, she is gradually realizing that the pain may always accompany her. She wonders whether it is possible to come to terms with the painful life, recently encouraged by Dr Jamesson, who insisted that she is actually a very strong person.

Introduction

Halvard Nilsen and Alice Kvale

A patient-centered approach is highly desirable when treating patients with CMP syndromes. The medical model should be replaced by a biopsychosocial model, thereby acknowledging that psychosocial features may be more important risk factors for chronicity and disability than biomedical symptoms and signs. In order to make adequate recommendations for rehabilitation it is necessary to recognize the patient's physical signs and symptoms, as well as her psychological, social and cultural background. The concept of 'Understanding the whole person' is an excellent tool for enhancing a clinical setting where the patient may give information of a social, emotional, cognitive and physical nature. The results of this phase of treatment guide both the patient and the health professional in finding common ground for the further process of recovery. By strengthening the patients' self-confidence and their ability to gain control over their own lives, the muscle-tonus and pain severity can be reduced.

Because of the non-specific criteria and the many different theories of cause(s) for CMP, a comprehensive and integrated biopsychosocial understanding may help us to explain the development and maintenance of the disease in the individual patient. The model of patient-centered medicine may also facilitate an understanding of how the pain syndrome in a particular patient is interwoven with other bodily expressions. This differs from the approach in some other patients, where the pathophysiology is often well understood. Many doctors still have to understand and experience the power of the method when working with such complex syndromes.

Evidence-based guidelines

For approximately the last decade, evidence-based guidelines for treatment have been published to assist both the practitioner and the patient to make decisions about appropriate treatment. Guidelines should reflect current knowledge at the time of publication, but the scientific rationale for the guidelines may be shortlived. Scientific advancements in medical, technical and psychological areas change the knowledge base, and hence the guidelines of treatment (Nordin and Campello, 1999). Within the treatment modalities for myofascial pain there is also a dilemma between experience-based knowledge and so-called evidence-based knowledge. Outcome studies and randomized controlled trials have become the gold standard for examining the efficiency of treatment. Knowledge of the effect of many treatment modalities based on controlled studies is still limited. A large number of available studies on the management of myofascial pain have methodological flaws. Patients with myofascial pain constitute a heterogenous group, and possible treatment effects for one patient sub-group may not be visible when several groups with different characteristics are pooled together (Bjordal and Greve, 1998). There are often discrepancies in treatment recommendations, and there also exists a gap between scientific evidence and the actual practice in clinical medicine. Guidelines based on evidence from systematic reviews are important to enhance our knowledge, but evidence-based medicine requires new skills, including efficient literature searching and the application of formal rules for evidence in evaluating the literature. Even today it must be accepted that our treatment modalities are based mainly on empiric grounds, and that new knowledge is strongly needed.

The consultation

A patient presenting with diffuse musculoskeletal symptoms, with secondary or many vague symptoms, may be vulnerable and afraid of being misunderstood. Some practitioners may have limited knowledge of dealing with such patients, and may meet the patient with attitudes influenced by morality, uncertainty or indignity. In order to show the patient respect, it is necessary to have an interest in the patient, to be polite, to listen before drawing conclusions and question if the conclusions fit with the patient's views. If the practitioner tries to get only objective information to fit into a disease-based model of thinking, there is a danger that the patient will also join 'the game of objectiveness'. Certainly, there are patients who will only gain confidence from the disease perspective, but it is important to clarify early that the practitioner is ready to listen and learn from the illness experience.

From treatment to rehabilitation

Many practitioners claim that it is very difficult to shift from consultations where the aim is to cure, to consultations with new content and methods in a setting where the first strategy has failed. In some sense, the doctor has not managed his/her first and primary goal; to cure the symptoms. This may give him or her a weakened position towards the patient. Will the patient still have confidence in her/him, although he/she has failed? It is not unreasonable that the patient may want a second opinion, or ask for a referral to a specialist. Many questions and expectations may not be resolved in open discussion.

Our advice in this situation would be to concentrate on building a new strategy together with the patient. A new hectic phase, with many referrals, cannot be recommended. The practitioner must re-evaluate the problems and revise all the information available. Why did the first strategy fail? The original acute pain has usually become a chronic pain syndrome at this stage. There are data showing that withdrawal from activities in the acute phase increases the risk for development of chronic pain (Epping-Jordan et al., 1998). The patient should therefore be encouraged to be active and to take responsibility for changes in life as early as possible.

Table 6.1 *Stages of change and therapist's tasks*

Patient's stage	Clinician's motivational tasks
Precontemplation	Raise doubt: increase the client's perception of the risks and problems associated with the current behavior.
Contemplation	Tip the balance: evoke reasons for change, risks of not changing, strengthen the client's self-efficacy for change of current behavior.
Preparation	Help the client to determine the best course of action.
Action	Help the client to take steps towards change.
Maintenance	Review progress; renew motivation and commitment as needed.
Relapse	Help the client review the processes of contemplation, determination and action, without becoming stuck or demoralized because of relapse.

Adapted from Miller and Rollnick (1991)

The clinician should inform the patient about relevant therapies, the mechanisms of action and data which demonstrate clinical efficacy. Providing patients with such information may enhance patient participation in decision-making and create more realistic expectations regarding treatment and rehabilitation outcomes. Finding common ground for the treatment plan needs a mutual understanding of emotions, expectations and medical thinking.

A cognitive approach is not only a therapeutic modality, but also a manner of communication and way of understanding the whole situation. According to this method it can be important to elucidate the patient's motivation for several tasks (e.g. home exercises, sleep hygiene, medication and challenge of the pain). Table 6.1 shows a motivational working plan during a process of change.

The social context of the chronic pain sufferer

In order to customize the treatment strategy, the physician must focus on stressors in the individual patient. The illness often has a special social consequence that bothers the patient more than the doctor is aware. Examples of such stressors may be an agreement to look after the grandchildren several days a week, that the employer will not accept a reduction in special work demands, a husband's lack of interest in the household, unsatisfactory sex-life, withdrawal from social activities or lack of documentation of functional loss for insurance purposes. In many patients, it is possible to find one special, important area of worry that may cause bad nights' sleep, powerlessness, depression or reinforcement of muscular pain. If such areas of concern are not detected, otherwise appropriate medical therapy may not help. Detection of such problems may reduce symptoms due to improved coping. Social strategy intervention (Roy, 1992) is based on advocacy, social support in the home and by friends and self-help groups. It may have a significant effect on the situation. A task-centered approach (Reid, 1978) can also be a powerful supportive method, with a focus on helping patients define their problems and find imaginative ways to resolve them.

Some factors that may guide the choice of therapy

Chronic pain syndromes are complex to treat, and treatment may be extensive and require many resources. A systematic evaluation is therefore important before making a treatment plan. Pain drawings, visual analogue scales for symptoms, inventories on health-related quality of life and mood states are all helpful and might be used. All kinds of information increase the understanding of the situation. The patient will often feel confident with such mapping activities. The data material can be directly used in the discussion on finding common ground, and to prioritize which of many symptoms is most important at the time.

The doctor should be aware of the risk of the patient adhering to a medical understanding of the symptoms. Medicalization may develop as a result of a physician's caring and long-time follow-up, including the prescribing of long-term medication. Medicines that can cure the disease are seldom available in myofascial pain. Medication that gives symptom relief can often be advised at some time. On the other hand, uncertainty about diagnosis, fear of having a malignancy or a progressive neurological or rheumatological disease may induce medicalization.

Both history-taking and the data from the clinical examination help to detect the main factors needing specific management. Some empirically based suggestions are listed below.

- Cognitive ability should be assessed. Sleep disorders and side effects from drugs should be focused on.
- Local or focal symptoms may need specific re-evaluation. Have relevant specialists been involved?

- Young adults should be examined for relative overload in their workplace. If the physical demands are out of the patient's capacity, strengthening exercises may help, but reoccurrence of symptoms will usually happen.
- A young adult who has never managed the demands of adult life may have unresolved hidden problems from youth or childhood.
- In the case of family sickness, think of learned illness. Is there psychiatric disease in the family, especially depressive disorders?
- Pain beliefs and patient's view on prognosis must be explored.
- Depression must be assessed carefully.
- An exact diagnosis of the type of pain should be sought. Psychogenic pain may be present. Severe function-loss because of pain in a person with no clinical signs and concomitant denial of any psychological or social problems is suspicious, and the patient should be referred, preferably to a multidisciplinary pain clinic.
- Somatization is common. The physician should explain possible consequences if medical help-seeking is out of proportion to the symptoms. The patient should be informed about somatoform disorders.
- Careful elucidation of any sexual problems can give useful information about the main problems that need treatment.
- If surgery is considered, conservative treatment modalities should have been tried first. There are often small differences in outcome after conservative and operative treatment for diseases like spinal stenosis, osteochondrosis, shoulder tendinosis and instability, lumbar disc herniation and cervicobrachialgia, but surgery may have irreversible complications.
- 'Burn-out syndrome', asthenia, loss of energy and chronic fatigue may be difficult to distinguish from depression.

Medication and injections

Halvard Nilsen

Despite extensive research with new understanding of pain-modulating mechanisms, there is a large gap between basic science and the tools available to the practitioner. There should be differences in approach to medication in the chronic pain setting compared with that of acute pain. The high prevalence rates of major depression, anxiety syndromes, substance and alcohol abuse and personality disorders in the group of patients with chronic pain may influence the treatment strategy. Pre-existing vulnerability may give more functional loss and worsen the prognosis. There may be individual responses to medical treatment, both positive and negative.

Box 6.1   *Drugs groups for the treatment of chronic pain disorders*

- Mild analgesics
- NSAIDs
- Opioids
- Antidepressants
- Anticonvulsants
- Muscle-relaxants
- Anxiolytics
- Injections

Long-lasting medical therapy should always be accompanied by a follow-up plan. The plan should be aimed at restoration of functions. Medication that does not bring pain relief or enhance activity should be discontinued, otherwise the medical therapy may be a negative factor because of adverse effects and negative cognitive strategies. Because of the multifactorial etiology, it is often necessary to try several modalities on the individual patient. The patient's own preferences should also be taken into account. In this text several different drugs are discussed (Box 6.1).

Mild analgesics

Mild analgesics such as aspirin and paracetamol/acetaminophen can offer moderate relief, and give additive effects when combined both with other drugs in this drug group and with drugs from other groups.

Non-steroidal anti-inflammatory drugs (NSAIDs)

Non-steroidal anti-inflammatory drugs can be helpful in pain states of mainly nociceptive origin and mild-to-moderate intensity. They can be combined with other medications, but are usually not effective in syndromes with symptoms of emotional distress. The best results will be achieved if the patient takes daily dosages without waiting for the pain to reach its maximum threshold. Some patients benefit from periodic use of these drugs, mainly in periods of high pain levels. The drugs have a ceiling effect, meaning that increasing the dosages beyond a certain threshold does not increase analgesia. Many patients do not continue using these drugs, mainly due to common adverse effects.

Opioids

The use of opioids in chronic non-malignant pain states is widely disputed in Western medicine (Portenoy, 1996). There are concerns about addiction, tolerance, persistent side effects and compromising both physical and psychosocial functioning. Cognitive and coping abilities in 'opioid patients' may be greatly reduced. Outcome studies of long-term therapy are limited, especially those describing the patient's overall situation when therapy is given for more than one year.

Most physicians should co-operate with a pain clinic if opioids (mostly morphine, oxycodone or methadone) are considered for non-malignant chronic pain states. All doctors are encouraged to comply with any existing national guidelines for treatment and follow-up of such patients.

Myofascial pain syndromes often do not respond well to opioid therapy. However, in Europe, codeine will often be prescribed initially, eventually in combination with non-opioid analgesics. If weak opioids are used in increasing dosages, the doctor must decide if he or she should continue this medication, make a reduction or shift to a trial of strong opioids. A trial with strong opioids may lead to concern for the doctor, the patient or the patient's family. Such therapy also needs a close follow-up, and much time will be used on drug-related factors.

Antidepressants

Tricyclic antidepressants (TCA) are effective for painful conditions, and they are generally well tolerated. A low dose of TCA (e.g. amitriptyline 10–90 mg) may have a positive effect on sleep and anxiety states. However, these drugs may have side effects which are mostly dose-dependent. When treating depressed or suicidal patients, toxicity must be considered. As a rule, it is advisable to try these drugs for a period of time, because of the very good results in some patients. But do not continue this medication if there are severe side effects or doubt about the effect.

Other antidepressants (like SSRIs) are not so useful for pain states, but may be used for depressive disorders or anxiety. There should be discussion with the patient, who should be well informed, as some patients do not experience or accept their coexisting disorder. Some are very vulnerable when not being understood regarding their somatic complaints.

Anticonvulsants

These agents are under continous evaluation and development for use in pain states. The neurogenic origin of both chronic pain and myofascial pain syndromes is probably common. The anticonvulsants reduce repetitive discharge and stabilize pain-transmitting cells. Carbamazepine, clonazepam and gabapentin are the most used agents, and can be given at low doses, titrated upward at set intervals. Effects and side effects should be monitored. Gabapentin is an especially interesting agent; relatively high doses seem to be well tolerated and give good pain relief in selected patients.

Muscle-relaxants

These drugs are mostly sedatives. They have many side effects and should therefore not be used for long-lasting therapy. Some patients take these drugs in order to obtain mental relaxation, but that seldom enhances rehabilitation strategies. Hidden anxiety states can be the reason for the pain in some patients, but these should be handled more appropriately.

Anxiolytics

In some individuals anxiolytics will give pain relief. Anxiety states associated with pain should, however, be treated by other therapeutic modalities, e.g. relaxation techniques or psychotherapy. Some patients may profit from low-dose tricyclic antidepressants or SSRIs.

Injections

Many studies have shown that trigger-point injections may have a positive effect on pain in patients with chronic pain. Injections may also stretch muscle and tendon tissue and induce long-standing improvement of function (Ashburn and Staats, 1999). Both dry-needling and local anesthetics may be used. Use of corticosteroids is not advised. Intramuscular stimulation (IMS) is a technique which combines elements of injection and acupuncture (Chan, 1996). The primary care physician can easily learn the technique.

A step aside: what could have happened to Judith Smith?

In this section we present a possible alternative course for Judith Smith, including a suggested four-session project with a shift in attitude to her problems.

On her next visit, Judith Smith's doctor told her that he had discussed her case with a colleague. This Dr Jones had great experience with chronic pain patients, and had offered to meet her and try to bring a new perspective to the negative situation both the doctor and the patient were experiencing. An appointment was already made for the same day, and Mrs Smith agreed to take part.

The first meeting was a discussion between the patient and the two doctors. Dr Jones told her that he had met several patients presenting similar symptoms, and that after several months many of them had obtained a better life. He proposed a process which included four sessions (once a week). The aim was to clarify her situation and introduce some new perspectives in order to make her function better. Her own doctor should step aside during this period, and just help her with other health problems, if necessary. He would be invited to the fourth session, to be brought back up to speed and help plan further management. It was suggested that Judith's husband should attend the third session.

Already, in the first session Judith felt confident with Dr Jones and the 'project'. The doctor presented a summary of what he understood about her situation from his discussions with her doctor and from reading her files. She was invited to discuss and correct his understanding. They communicated in a way that also gave Judith insight into new ways of seeing her own situation. She got a strong feeling of being understood, her symptoms were focused on and she realized that she was not alone with these types of pain.

Dr Jones mentioned how partners with grown-up children had different coping strategies for problems in their marriage. Some did not talk about the future at all, but just felt that something was wrong and that they spent less and less time together. Judith could very well see that this was the situation in her own marriage. She now wanted to have her own life with her husband, but could not always interpret his feelings for her. He was often away from home at evenings and weekends. She felt how talking about this to the doctor made her afraid and depressed, and she also felt how her muscles cramped and gave her a headache when she did.

In the second session, Dr Jones did an extensive clinical examination. He explained his findings. He had found sore, non-elastic and short musculature in her neck and shoulder region and her upper body as a whole, very typical for patients with a stressful and demanding life. He also found a myotendinitis in her left buttock, which was treated by an injection with anesthetic and corticosteroid. Dr Jones told her that this kind of muscular symptom was typical in individuals who made heavy demands on themselves. Judith felt that this was a precise description of her own situation. Other topics that were discussed were her job situation and her private economy. Her husband was willing to meet Dr Jones.

Dr Jones did not want to give her antidepressant medication. She felt that was a right decision. She told Dr Jones that she had felt more depressed than she had told her own doctor, because she didn't want to be forced to use antidepressants.

During the third session, Judith's husband got the opportunity to describe how he had seen his wife grow more and more desperate, and how this had made himself depressed and dysfunctional in the role of a husband. He was informed about how demands and stress could be important factors in pain syndromes, and that it is possible to stop negative processes and thus get better. They both were told that she might not be as strong physically as in her youth, but could have a much better life. They responded positively to achieving this goal. Dr Jones suggested some possible steps in order to reduce pain and improve her functioning. He wanted them to discuss them and the consequences there would be at home. Judith should present their conclusions at the fourth session, and a plan should be set thereafter. She was given a leaflet about therapy with low-dose antidepressants for myofascial pain and sleep disorders.

The fourth session started with Judith and Dr Jones updating her own doctor, and the discussion ended with the formulation of a plan.

- Work demands would be reduced by taking one day off every week for at least six months. The day would be used to do *some* housework.
- She would start low-intensity physical training twice a week; Wednesday and Sunday. A physiotherapist would develop a protocol and follow-up her progress. Judith was told that she might feel more pain and exhaustion in the first few weeks, but gradually she would feel better. She should do the Sunday training sessions with her husband.
- She was advised to start with amitriptyline; 10 mg two hours before sleep, eventually increasing the dosage to 25 mg.
- Her husband would do the housework with her on Saturdays. He would also stay at home more evenings.
- Judith would consult her doctor once a month at first, and also have contact with Dr Jones and the physiotherapist. Her husband would meet them with her at least every third month.

Six months later the doctors and the physiotherapist met to discuss the situation. They summarised: Judith felt stronger, had more energy, had lost several pounds in weight and felt more fit. Her husband did more of the housework, and he was more interested in spending time with her. They had more insight into common afflictions, and were determined to go on together. Their sexual life was better. She had some pain relief after starting with the antidepressants, and she used TENS several times a day. The doctors agreed that her life seemed to be developing constructively, and that only monthly follow-up was needed. Judith and her husband felt that the doctors had a good understanding of what was happening.

Modifying the frame of patient–physician interaction, exemplified by writing an illness diary

Per Stensland

The patient–physician relationship may be supported and facilitated by special communication tools (Malterud, 1992). Some authors recommend the use of written material from the patient as a means to grasp the thoughts, feelings and ideas connected with the symptoms. Recent studies indicate that a change in the use of words in personal-illness narratives may predict an improvement in health (Pennebaker *et al.*, 1997) and that writing about stressful events can improve symptoms in chronic disease (Pennebaker, 2000; Smyth *et al.*, 1999).

Inviting the patient to formulate an illness diary in writing is one way of giving the patient and the physician access to the illness narrative, providing a supplementary channel for communication and enhancing the presentation of symptoms in the patient's own language. In a qualitative study on consultations with 16 patients suffering from long-standing illness without clinical findings, Stensland and Malterud focused on how the use of an illness diary affects the verbal interaction in general practice consultations (Stensland & Malterud, 1997, 1999), by giving access to the patient's own metaphors.

The following is a presentation of the use of illness diaries as a clinical method intended for information collection and as an intervention in family practice consultations.

The illness diary

The clinical method

The illness diary method is more a flexible approach to patient–physician inter-action than a fixed technical procedure. The physician's introductory remark could be:

'Do you think this might be useful to explore in writing?

Here you have a sheet of paper. I would recommend you make notes about your illness. Do you have any idea how to shape it? . . . If not, my previous patients have given me these cues . . .'

The patient may choose to make free diary notes on a blank sheet of paper, or utilize a structured format. The structured diary sheet is meant to register symp-tom information along one axis and date/time along the other. The columns have no fixed headings, but are supposed to be labeled, as the dialogue indicates items for further inquiry. The patient's own terms should preferably be used to describe these items and serve as headings for the columns. Initially, these may be the patient's expressions for the symptom, its strength, localization, dura-tion, accompanying complaints and an open column for comments. The patient returns after three to four weeks, and the physician reads the notes while the patient listens (Figure 6.1).

The subsequent conversation may identify additional items for further dia-logue. These may concern bodily changes or still-unclarified somatic complaints. This procedure may deepen the patient's first symptom presentation, in a way that starts with, and gradually introduces, a change in the clinical dialogue.

Patients may not be used to thinking of days or periods when they were 'normal' or not suffering. The illness diary may be used to identify and charac-terize days when the symptoms are partly reduced.

The diaries may also deal with relational issues: who was present at the onset of symptoms, who was able to help, and what did help. Relational questions, which patients may feel are provocative when presented alone, may be more easily appreciated by the patients when integrated in a broader context. The physician's invitation to this dialogue on contextual issues may be:

'When you have written this, and you get an overview of it, what kind of ideas do you get about it?'

The dialogues following from the diary notes demonstrate how perception of bodily symptoms may be accompanied by negative thoughts. Such accompany-ing ideas, expressed as repetitive, pessimistic 'internal voices', can be elucidated

Name: Judith Smith

DATE	ILLNESS	WHEN, HOW	OTHER COMPLAINT	MEDICATION	COMMENTS
2/2	Chestpain	Not so bad today After work		–	
4/2	Pain in chest and left arm	Worse than yesterday	Headache	1 tablet	Too busy day
5/2	Tingling feeling left arm			–	Anna started a quarrel
8/2	Chest pain and pain in neck	Woke up with pain	Headache	2 tablets	This pain is creeping around every muscle
9/2	Left part of my chest		Nausea, palpitation	1 tablet	

Figure 6.1   Illness diary of Judith Smith, based on the case in Chapter 3.

through the illness diary. The physician's invitation to a discussion on internal dialogues may be:

'When experiencing symptoms or pain, people may hear themselves saying something, or an idea may come to mind. Have you experienced anything like that? Would it be possible to write down what these internal voices say?'

Diaries as interactional frames

The distinction between open (a blank sheet of paper) or structured format of the illness diary may be important for some patients' participation. A flexible format, open for negotiation between physician and patient, may make it suitable for the individual. From a search for a device to help the physician know 'what to do' in the encounter, more emphasis should be put on how to co-operate in this field. Inviting the patient to discuss how to talk about her/his problem is an extension of the ambition to let the patient's concepts and descriptions frame the medical dialogue.

The physician may experience that diary notes may be scarce and compressed, but some patients may produce more elaborate reports. However, even brief notes may enable a fresh and productive frame for conversation.

New ideas

For the patient, writing an illness diary may introduce new ideas for discussion at the next consultation. The diary may act as an extension of a short consultation, with topics having been discussed expanding into the patient's life. The patient may document his/her discussions with parents, spouse or children about the illness.

The physician may also change his attitude to the patient and to the ensuing encounter, as the additional contextual information presents the patient more clearly as a whole person. The physician may positively anticipate being presented with material that is previously unknown to him or her, instead of going through a repetition of other sessions. Thus, the illness diary may help him/her be more inquisitive and thus reinforce a positive attitude to the conversation.

Limitations

Any communicative method may be regarded as manipulative by increasing the physician's power. The clinical method presented here, however, is intended to empower patients by balancing the input from physician and patient in the medical dialogue.

Diaries do not suit everybody. Some patients may feel the method does not appeal to them after being introduced to it. The physician may get the impression that they lack the curiosity needed to search for more information. In other cases, he/she may feel she/he knows the patient so well that there is no need for further information collection.

The diary: a slow and silent conversation

Some authors have recommended three elements in the consultation with patients suffering from chronic pain: show understanding, help with a fresh approach to the symptoms and help to see connections between symptoms and life. The illness narrative presented to the physician is one of several possible ways of telling a personal story. In order to explore the story, it needs to be expressed openly or privately. By means of writing, a person extends the internal dialogue by testing it out first on paper. A slow and silent conversation takes place. Formulating sensitive matters in writing can help the patient recognize hidden aspects of their illness, while the process of externalization creates a sense of distance from inherent emotional pain. This is exemplified by Peter, the 36-year-old man (*see* Chapter 3) who related differently to his problems when they were written down. The transition from spoken word to written text seems to clarify the person's relationship to the matter.

The French philosopher Paul Ricoeur claims that writing is a way of fixing fluent speech (Ricoeur, 1971). Once written down, the connection between the meaning of a word and the speaker's emotional response to it is broken. The written statement may acquire a feeling of distance or objectivity, as it is released from the subjective intention of the writer. The written text starts an independent life, ready to be freshly interpreted by anyone, including the writer. This transformation of speech into text generates a surplus of meaning from a creative distance.

The intimate nature of spoken dialogue may not only open, but can also close down communication. Ricoeur holds that the written text, by introducing the aspect of distance, has the ability to negotiate tacit and basic aspects of a joint language, which may be overheard in fluent speech. Writing diary notes may create a clarifying distance from the patient's illness experience. When writing is part of a purposeful activity intended to elucidate a specific dilemma, the person may establish a self-administered observant position or metaposition in relation to his or her own problem.

Cross-disciplinary approaches and physiotherapy

Alice Kvale and Lucy M Candib

The foundation for choice of treatment is based on a close relationship between the data acquired during a thorough assessment phase, and the nature, focus and goals of the therapeutic regimen. Three key questions need to be addressed through anamnestic conversation and physical evaluation, independent of which discipline the health person represents:

1 What is wrong?
2 How did it develop?
3 What can be done?

Individual predisposing and perpetuating risk factors for the myofascial pain problems need to be acknowledged within many areas. Examples of physical predisposing and/or perpetuating risk factors are de-conditioning, relative muscle strength, decreased mobility, muscular tension, sleep problems, repetitive overuse of arms and heavy work combined with poor physical fitness and tiredness.

In managing pain, the clinician should inform the patient about relevant therapies, the known mechanism of action and data demonstrating clinical efficacy, if available. Providing patients with such information may enhance patient participation in decision-making and create more realistic expectations regarding treatment outcome.

A cognitive–behavioral approach

In the last few years, there has been increasing focus on the role that cognitive and affective factors have in the patient's perception of how to deal with pain. Therapeutic gain is allegedly enhanced and only maintained when the patient is actively involved, accepts responsibility for change and is intrinsically motivated rather than externally manipulated. The specific techniques employed in treatment are of less significance. A cognitive–behavioral approach should be present in the following treatment modalities. The cognitive–behavioral approach can be adapted for use with inpatients and outpatients, conducted on an individual or group basis and used as a total program for treatment for chronic pain patients in a multidisciplinary setting, or by a set of solo practitioners from specific disciplines (Turk and Rudy, 1994).

Specific treatment: complementary therapies

Specific treatment interventions for systemic or regional long-lasting myofascial pain generally include techniques or modalities such as those listed in Table 6.2. These interventions can be used alone or in combination. The foundations for practice are drawn from theory, research, tradition and belief. However, contradiction for use is still found in the literature dealing with treatment of long-lasting myofascial pain.

Physical modalities

These can be defined as the use of physical energy or agents in producing a therapeutic effect on pain modulation. The therapeutic objective is to provide symptomatic relief, and for some modalities, to reduce inflammation, muscular symptoms and joint stiffness. The agents and modalities include heat, ice, laser treatment, electrical stimulation, TENS and hydrotherapy.

Table 6.2   Specific treatment interventions for systemic or regional myofascial pain

Physical modalities	Heat, ice, electrical stimulation, laser treatment, TENS, hydrotherapy
Manual techniques	Different soft tissue mobilization techniques such as local or whole-body massage, direct pressure, myofascial release, muscle energy techniques, manual stretch, etc.
Exercise training	Therapeutic exercises, including different regimes such as medical exercise therapy (MET), McKenzie, Kraus exercise program, etc.
Relaxation programs	Autogenic training, transcendental meditation or yoga, Jacobson's method of progressive relaxation, stress management training, etc. Biofeedback treatment
Manipulation therapy	A variety of diagnostic and therapeutic manual techniques from manipulation (with high velocity thrust) to mobilization (no thrust)

Physical modalities are popular for many reasons, including the patient's expectations of traditional physical therapy and the satisfaction of not having to exert themselves. When used as the only treatment, passive modalities are, however, much discussed as there seems to be sparse evidence of their actual effect, especially long-term, on musculoskeletal pain problems. They can be employed to decrease pain prior to conditioning and restorative activities. Physical modalities are usually better than no treatment, but not always more efficacious than placebo. Those patients who receive a variety of forms of therapy seem to do best (Feine and Lund, 1997). Physical agents should only be used in combination with exercise and movement retraining, and discontinued if positive effects are not apparent within a few treatment sessions (8–10). Furthermore, a transition to home techniques should be made as quickly as possible. As the effect of passive modalities is mainly temporary relief, the best option may be to teach the patient self-application of heat, cold or TENS if pain reduction is demonstrated in the individual. It is important to insure that the use of passive modalities does not inactivate the patient or reinforce his/her sick role (Sheon et al., 1996).

One recent study showed that chronic low back pain patients who received individually adapted conventional physical therapy (heat or cold, massage, stretching, different forms of electrotherapy, traction and a few exercises on the treatment table) obtained significantly better results concerning pain, function, patient satisfaction and costs compared to patients who were left untreated (Torstensen et al., 1998).

Manual techniques

Included in manual therapies are soft tissue mobilization techniques such as massage (kneading, stroking, and rolling of muscles, skin and other soft tissues), direct pressure (ischemic pressure or myotherapy as a means to deactivate tender points or pain points), myofascial release (mobilization of soft tissue, focusing on fascial planes as well as muscle tissue), muscle energy techniques (a blend of manual techniques and guided muscle contractions to affect changes in alignment and muscle performance and to correct motion dysfunction), and manual stretch to tender/trigger points (direct mechanical stretch to tissues that may be preceded or accompanied by use of a spray that chills the area). The practitioner's sense of touch is central, and tactile sensation is the avenue of communication between patient and practitioner. Massage is outlined in some detail below.

Manual techniques in their various forms have been offered for centuries as methods for relieving pain. It is still somewhat uncertain what pain condition will respond best to which treatment. As with most treatment techniques mentioned in this chapter, this is seldom offered on its own, but as part of a larger regimen.

Whole-body massage therapy

Whole-body massage therapy is an approach to CMP that can be classified under physiotherapy, supportive therapy or complementary therapy. Massage therapy is considered a 'supportive' treatment because the goal of the massage therapist is to support pain relief and relaxation. In most countries, massage remains a 'complementary' therapy peripheral to mainstream medicine. It is often regarded as a 'New Age frill' or a luxury, and not a treatment regimen in its own right.

Whole-body massage therapy involves the manipulation of deep tissues, stimulating pressure receptors, stretching muscles, breaking up adhesions and increasing blood flow. In a randomized comparison study of massage therapy for fibromyalgia, two 30-minute massage treatments per week for five weeks were compared with TENS, and sham TENS. The patients receiving massage reported less anxiety and depression, had greater relief of pain, less stiffness and fatigue and fewer interrupted nights (Sunshine *et al.*, 1997). Massage therapy has also demonstrated efficacy in the treatment of migraines, low back pain, depression, anxiety, PTSD, and CFS (Field, 1998).

Massage therapy may be both an appropriate and useful treatment for CMP as well as for medically unexplained disorders. Massage therapy has a direct effect of promoting lengthening of contracted and tensed muscles, with an immediate, resulting relaxation both at the local and general body level. Repeated treatments within a short period, such as four to eight weeks, offer the possibility of maintaining these gains from one treatment to the next, and decreasing overall pain over time. Massage therapy also promotes whole-body relaxation that is often unavailable to people with chronic pain syndromes. Such relaxation promotes better sleep, helping to break the cycle of pain and sleeplessness. Massage therapy addresses the place that hurts. The therapist touches the pain. The importance of touch itself in healing, though infrequently studied, cannot be overestimated. For some chronic pain patients, especially women, massage may be the only form of non-sexual, non-abusive touch in their life. For patients who have suffered prior physical abuse either as children or adults, chronic pain may directly and indirectly relate to the injuries and fear and tension associated with those injuries. Massage therapy may address such 'body memories'.

The whole-body massage treatment takes the whole person into account; it is founded on the assumption that there is a connection between pains in various parts of the body. Massage therapy thus supports the patient's experience of herself as a whole person suffering in connected ways, rather than as a collection of assorted, unrelated pains, as she appears in the biomedical model.

Exercise training

This can be defined as a series of specific movements for the purpose of training or developing the body through systematic practice, or as a bodily exertion for the promotion of physical health. The goal can be to prevent and reduce pain, to gain strength, flexibility and endurance, to restore injured tissues, and to promote activities of daily living. Therapeutic exercises are supervised and the tempo and load of the exercise can be controlled and adjusted by the therapist as well as by the patient. Some exercise techniques have specific regimes, e.g. the Kraus exercise program (Wyszynski, 1997), the McKenzie method (Simonsen, 1998), or medical exercise therapy (MET) (Torstensen *et al.*, 1998). Exercises can also be more general and performed outside therapy rooms, in gymnasiums, in indoor or outdoor sports leisure centers, at the workplace, at home, etc.

The focus of exercise for patients with myofascial pain is primarily directed at preventing impairments, functional limitations and disabilities, not at a tissue-level healing process. It is, however, difficult to define the exact content of exercises, and to compare exercise with other treatment modalities. The patient's motivation to perform exercise can be influenced by many factors, internal (motivation) as well as external (social and financial hinders/awards). The questions of 'to whom, why, when, how, how long and how often' are open for further research.

A recent randomized controlled trial documented that exercise (high-intensity progressive–resistive training for large muscle groups, three days a week for 10 weeks) improved subjective sleep quality and significantly reduced depression (Singh *et al.*, 1997). Exercise also plays a part in the patients' physical and psychological abilities to return to work. Exercise combined with behavioral management or workplace intervention achieves better results than exercise alone (Linton, 1994).

The exercise programs chosen will vary depending on type and duration of pain problem(s). Exercise programs that commence after six weeks of non-specific back pain have been reported to yield a superior clinical outcome when compared with other treatments (Nordin and Campello, 1999). Fibromyalgia patients can undertake an exercise program which includes aerobic, flexibility and strength training exercises without adverse effects, and with significant results, including decrease in tender points and increase in fitness (Martin *et al.*, 1996). Positive long-term effects for patients with fibromyalgia seems, however, dependent on adherence to an exercise program with relative high intensity over time (30–45 minutes at least three times per week for >12 weeks) (Wigers *et al.*, 1996). It seems preferable for patients with long-lasting myofascial pain to combine exercise with coping skills training, including relaxation (Sandstrom and Keefe, 1998). It cannot be sufficiently stressed that treatment programs must be individually adapted. In other words, one has to bear in mind that patients with fibromyalgia are a heterogeneous group. For some, exercises with high intensity will be too strenuous and pain-provoking. Treatment with low-intensity exercises, with focus on body-awareness techniques and coping, might then be the best choice.

Relaxation and meditation programs

Standardized instructions or meditative techniques are used to elicit a relaxation response, characterized by generalized decreases in the sympathetic nervous system and metabolic activity and an altered state of consciousness, described as a subjective experience of well-being. The techniques include autogenic training (patients are taught to achieve feelings of heaviness and warmth in their limbs), transcendental meditation or yoga (deep relaxation accompanied by subjective experiences of 'peace of mind and a sense of well-being') and Jacobson's method of progressive relaxation (people are taught to relax individual muscle groups in progression) (Benson *et al.*, 1977; Jacobson, 1987).

Relaxation training, often combined with coping skills training and stress management, may be a central part of the treatment of long-lasting myofascial pain problems, but should be used in addition to exercise, not alone (Martin *et al.*, 1996; Sandstrom and Keefe, 1998). Review of several stress management studies shows that relaxation and behavioral skills are helpful and that group methods are both more cost-effective and more beneficial than individual counseling (Sims, 1997). In a few studies, relaxation techniques are compared with other forms of conservative treatments. In one small study, chronic low back pain patients were randomly assigned to three treatment conditions. Eight sessions with relaxation training, consisting of progressive relaxation, breathing techniques, autogenic training and visual imagery, gave better results in reducing EMG and pain and increasing relaxation and activity than either EMG biofeedback alone or a placebo condition (Stuckey *et al.*, 1986). Stress management treatment can have beneficial short-term effect on pain, tenderness and depression in patients with fibromyalgia, and better long-term compliance has been shown, compared with aerobic exercise (Wigers *et al.*, 1996).

Biofeedback treatment

With the help of sensitive electronic equipment which monitors a person's EEG, heart rate, blood pressure or muscle tension, it has become possible to 'feed back' these biological signals to the person (visually or auditory) so that she knows, for example, that certain muscles are tense rather than relaxed. Then, the person can be better taught to relax to reduce muscle tension.

Biofeedback therapy research has shown that this is useful for relieving pain in some people. It can be a useful tool for distraction of attention, relaxation, suggestion and for providing the patient with a sense of control over their pain. In one recent RCT study of patients with fibromyalgia (n = 119) the effectiveness of three different forms of treatment, biofeedback (combined with relaxation training), exercise training and combination treatment, was compared with an educational/attention control group. All three treatment interventions resulted in improved self-efficacy for physical function, best maintained over time (two years) by the combination group (Buckelew *et al.*, 1998). However, most studies are small, and there are somewhat contradictory results, which pours doubt on whether biofeedback is a recommendable treatment method or not for patients with long-lasting pain problems. Quite a few studies concern patients with localized pain problems, such as either tension headache or myofascial pain of the temporomandibular joint. Biofeedback could be considered if there is muscle hyperactivity, fairly localized pain, and if there are few other problems, such as no depression. In patients with more generalized myofascial pain, general relaxation techniques without the use of expensive equipment seem to work just as well (Jessup and Gallegos, 1994).

Manipulation therapy and chiropractic

This includes a variety of manually performed techniques, often consisting of high velocity thrust procedures applied to a joint or series of joints and soft tissues. The procedures, generally performed by professionals, often physiotherapists with special training, chiropractors or osteopaths, are supposed to 'gap' or move the joint very quickly. Manipulations are carried out to create extra freedom of movement and to relieve pain.

There is disagreement over whether or not manipulation is a treatment of choice for patients with chronic pain. For low back pain patients with subacute pain, manipulation is recommended by some. If manipulation has not resulted in symptomatic and functional improvement after four weeks, it should be stopped and the patient re-evaluated. Long-term manipulation beyond this timeline has not been shown to be effective (Nordin and Campello, 1999; Waddell, 1998). Others have suggested that manipulation might be considered for chronic low back pain conditions that have lasted more than 12 weeks. For patients with neck pain and headache there is some evidence that spinal manipulation and mobilization probably provide some short-term benefits (Hurwitz *et al.*, 1996). However, as manipulation (with high velocity thrust) is no better than mobilization (with no thrust), the use of manipulation with high velocity thrust is cautioned. Manipulation, combined with exercise, can also have a role in treatment of localized problems, such as shoulder dysfunctions, but not for generalized myofascial pain problems (Sheon *et al.*, 1996).

Communication between physicians and physiotherapists

In most Western societies, primary care physicians manage most musculoskeletal problems. However, as both training in this area and consultation time available often is limited, some aspects of management may be suboptimal. When pain problems have become subacute and signs of delayed recovery are present (>4 weeks), there might be an advantage in cross-disciplinary co-operation. Physiotherapists should have qualifications to provide the primary care physicians with a thorough examination and a treatment proposal. Timing of intervention seems to be an important factor in rehabilitation of pain problems. Some studies indicate that physicians should request physiotherapy service early, i.e. within four to six weeks after injury or onset of pain problems. Patients who are referred early seem to return sooner to work than those who are referred later (Ehrmann-Feldman *et al.*, 1996).

Multidisciplinary treatment

There is increasing evidence that the choice of treatment for fibromyalgia and other chronic pain syndromes is multidisciplinary programs. Multidisciplinary treatments for chronic pain have been shown to be superior to no treatment, being held on a waiting list, or single-discipline treatments such as medical treatment or physical therapy. Findings from meta-analyses, review articles and recent clinical trials suggest that interventions that combine exercise and psychoeducational approaches designed to enhance communication, control, problem-solving and coping can have a clinically significant impact on reducing pain, improving emotional well-being and functional status for many conditions (Flor *et al.*, 1992; Værøy and Merskey, 1993).

Physiotherapy for Judith Smith?

She may be referred to a one to two-hour physiotherapy evaluation where both her bodily status and her working capacity should be evaluated. The physiotherapist should then share her conclusions with the doctor. After the patient has gone through a full evaluation giving information about her current condition, physically as well as psychosocially, the patient and the doctor can better contemplate how factors that perpetuate her problems can be addressed.

Based on the above-mentioned information about available treatment options, the doctor and the patient should decide on what might be optimal for Judith. Gauging how long she has had the problems is a central starting point. The doctor might be well aware of the difference in treatment options available when the pain problem is acute vs subacute or chronic, but rarely the patient. As Judith's problems has been long-lasting, referral to treatment with passive modalities should be ruled out with an explanation as to why. Exercises recommended earlier have not been completed, and she has, at this stage, no energy on her own to try again. A referral to a rehabilitation clinic for multidisciplinary treatment might give her a possibility to 'recharge her batteries'.

A multimodal management strategy with a cognitive–behavioral approach offers the greatest improvement potential for long-lasting pain syndromes. The combination of therapies may provide her with the skills and knowledge needed to increase her sense of control over pain. The integration of physiotherapy, psychological techniques, and, if necessary, appropriate pharmacotherapeutic regimens maximizes a patient's effectiveness in dealing with chronic pain. The doctor should also request that Judith should receive work-related evaluation and information during her treatment period.

From individual treatment to learning in groups: a group-learning program as an example of occupational rehabilitation approaches

Eldri Steen and Liv Haugli

Occupation and occupation-related factors influence the prevalence of CMP (Tsai *et al.*, 1992). There are many hypotheses concerning the relationship between working conditions and development of chronic pain. Work-related risk factors can be divided into physical and psychosocial groups. The physical stress factors commonly include heavy workload, static posture, frequent handling and twisting, heavy lifting, pushing, pulling, carrying, repetitive work and vibration. Psychosocial stress factors include high work pace, low level of control, little work support and low job satisfaction (Karasek and Theorell, 1990). This perspective calls for a wide assessment of ergonomic workplace design. Most ergonomic intervention programs modify the loads, the design of objects handled, lifting techniques, workplace layout and task design. The effectiveness of these interventions in controlling medical costs or morbidity has not been clearly demonstrated (Halpern, 1992), and it is proposed that ergonomic interventions alone may be sub-optimal in controlling myofascial problems (Burton *et al.*, 1997). More promising in this respect are programs that take into account the personal and interpersonal aspects influencing disability.

A number of behavioral and relaxation intervention programs exist, and are effective in the treatment of chronic pain (Goldenberg, 1993; NIH Technology Assessment Panel, 1996). In this chapter we describe a group-learning program based on personal construct theory which was carried out in an occupational health service setting.

Theoretical foundations and an expansion of the methodological repertoire: an example of an occupational health approach

This program has an integrating approach that includes a phenomenological understanding of the mind–body relationship. This implies that the myofascial complaints of the participant are not only seen in relation to ergonomic factors in their work situation, but as related to their whole-life situation.

A phenomenological perspective implies searching for the essence in the individual's experience. The lifeworld of each person has its own meaningful structure that needs to be approached in a way that is different from the natural sciences (Merleau-Ponty, 1996). Maurice Merleau-Ponty argues that a person's understanding of the world has its basis in her/his body's understanding of the situation and surroundings. The human body is thus not an object, but our center and carrier of experiences. We experience meaning directly in our bodies; people we have been connected to are both in us and with us, as much as time and places. Within this frame of understanding, CMP might be interpreted as a reaction, developed over years, to the totality of a person's life experiences, including workload and an ergonomically wrong working position.

Including a phenomenological approach presupposes willingness from occupational health personnel to expand their methodological repertoire when approaching employees with CMP. In addition to assessing ergonomic analysis, the occupational health service might also create possibilities for employees to become aware of possible relations between their bodily symptoms, emotions, mind and life situation.

This can be achieved by offering employees participation in a group-learning program based on the perspective presented above. An underlying assumption of such a program is that reconstruction of meaning is possible; we do not only construe experiences and situations to create meaning, but we are also able to reconstruct our interpretations and create new constructs (Kelly, 1955). A salutogenetic perspective where the employees' resources and potentials are focused on, rather than their pain and disability, is also essential. Special training in the use of creative teaching and counseling methods to enhance these perspectives and in handling group processes is a presupposition for working within this perspective. The training of health personnel must focus on the importance of not interpreting for participants, nor giving advice or presenting the 'right' answers, but rather to encourage each participant in becoming aware of and searching for possible meaning in her/his painful muscles. To operate within the participants' own language and ways of expressing themselves rather than using professional language ensures that the activities are based on the participants' own understanding. The many different methods and exercises to be used are thus based on a philosophy of teaching that acknowledges a participatory view of knowledge, an active relation between the learner and the subject matter and personal experiences as essential to learning.

The program

Working book

Each participant gets a working book that is to be used throughout the program. She/he is to take spontaneous notes on whatever comes to mind after an exercise in order to 'process' the experience while it is still vivid. This will enhance the participants' possibilities of becoming aware of what they have learned and how thoughts, feelings and bodily reactions can be related to the experience (Pennebaker *et al.*, 1987).

Metaphors

The program contains the use of metaphors, both the ones that are brought forward by the group members, and metaphors introduced by the occupational health personnel. The meaning of the metaphor is grounded within our experience and embedded in cultural assumptions, values and attitudes. Metaphors as mental structures are outside our conventional conceptual system, and are as such imaginative and creative. They are not only able to give new meaning to the past and to our daily activities, but they also have the power to create new reality if the metaphor becomes a deeper reality and the individual starts acting according to it.

Guided imagery

Guided imagery is a mental activity that makes it possible to 'travel' both in time and space, and to experience the wholeness of relationships and situations. Metaphors can be used as part of the guided imagery. Imagery is always personal and unique, and the meaning resides with the imager. The image might be experienced with all senses, offer new perspectives, temporarily suspend critical judgements and make anything possible. The images are embedded in each person's personal history and cultural background.

Crayons, paper and movement to different music

Aspects of our lives might not conform neatly to words because they are pre-verbal, but they might be expressed by colour, shape, movement and sound. Some exercises in the program use crayons and paper and movement to different music. The use of drawing contains two different processes: when the participant draws and when they use the drawing as self-instruction afterwards. The visual system and drawing can function independently of language, while the second phase is related to verbal processes. Movement to music offers possibilities of rediscovering the body by becoming aware of it, the mind and feelings in relation to 'opening up' to what the different music evokes and 'taking space' on the floor.

Sharing

Sharing with group members and group leaders after exercises and free writing might lead to two outcomes: firstly, the individual who takes the risk to disclose important personal feelings and thoughts acknowledges her/his own construction of knowledge and thus enhances self-awareness; secondly, others are able to see themselves in relation to the person whose history is told.

Awareness and mindful meditation

The participants are taught to pay attention to their breathing, mind and body. Paying attention to what happens inside requires practice. Mindful meditation allows you to learn from your own inner experience that pain is something you can work with, befriend, listen to and in some way, honour.

Each meeting has a theme, but no specific outcome is expected. Each participant is encouraged to work at her/his own 'speed', and participation in the different exercises is voluntary. The different methods described above are used at each session. Doing homework related to discoveries from participating in exercises and sharing between group members is part of the program. The themes of a program can be the following: 'If my body could talk . . .', strengthening of the self and inner voice through focusing on 'who am I?', 'what do I need?', awareness of 'humor, joy and laughter', 'guilt', 'anger', 'sorrow', possible differences between espoused values and values in use, awareness of resources, potentials and choices and strengthening of the 'road ahead'.

Short and long-term effects of the group-learning program

Effects of the group program, as described above, were tested in a randomized controlled study (Haugli *et al.*, 2000). Pain reduction was seen only at the one-year follow-up, whereas pain-coping abilities and abilities to cope with life demands were found to be improved immediately after the end of the program and maintained at follow-up (Haugli *et al.*, 2001). This may indicate that reconstruction and changing behavioral patterns that might influence pain take time, and that the learning program may have initiated this process of reconstruction. The participants also report increased awareness of self and others, and a change of focus towards a more positive outlook both in relation to pain and their life situation.

The evaluation of the intervention program further demonstrated reduced healthcare consumption, and this reduction was maintained at the follow-up. The rate of disability pension was also reduced. Absenteeism, however, did not seem to differ significantly from the control group. This may be due to the fact that more of those who participated in the intervention program were still in the workforce one year after the end of the program. Being a more marginal workforce, they had more sick leave.

Discussion

The described study does not provide empirical information on what elements of the intervention program provided pain reduction. The exercises offered intertwined and complemented each other. The aim was always to give participants possibilities to become aware and experience how emotions, cognition and life situation might influence bodily reactions. The same exercise did not necessarily give the same meaning to all participants, since pain and bodily meaning of pain is individual. Listening to other group participants may have helped them become aware of their own constructs, and experiencing how different reconstructions helped the other participants may have been an emotional support in their own reconstruction process.

This example of rehabilitation of CMP patients implies learning a new methodological repertoire for the occupational health personnel. Changing pain behavior and emotional patterns takes time as we see from the example of Judith Smith as she joins the group. The cost/benefit of the program may thus need further investigation.

There seem to be similarities between the described program and cognitive therapies, but there are also differences: neither the epistemology of contemporary cognitive psychology nor the phenomenological realm and the complex nature of lived human experience have been fully examined. An explicit awareness of the body as a 'talking' subject, with possible 'hidden' emotions, such as guilt, sadness and anger in painful muscles, might not be valid knowledge within a cognitive therapy frame of understanding.

The described program can be criticized for focusing too much on individual coping strategies at the expense of organizational factors. We stress, however, the importance of including ergonomic, organizational and individual aspects in the approach towards reducing myofascial pain in the workplace.

Judith Smith joins the group

In addition to making an ergonomic analysis of Judith Smith's work situation, the occupational health service of the hospital invites her to join a group-learning program for employees with CMP. The program will last for four hours each session, with a two-week interval between sessions. Participants will have to do some homework between sessions. Ten employees are invited to participate in the group.

Judith was sceptical from the start. She had not really understood what it meant to take part in a group process and possibly make new discoveries about her pain. Up until now the family physician was the one she had trusted even if he did not seem to be able to remove her pain. The two occupational health personnel, one a physician and one a nurse, acted differently in the group than the health personnel she was used to. Even though the group members were bound to secrecy, she did not like that some of them were also working in the hospital laundry.

After the first session, she was not sure that she wanted to continue. She had suddenly started crying when she participated in an exercise where she was supposed to sit still and become aware of different parts of her body, thoughts and feelings. She felt embarrassed. Some of the other participants had shared their reactions after exercises, but she had not liked listening to them. Participation in a relaxation exercise at the end of the session was a good experience, however, and she had felt less tension in her body for some hours afterwards.

As homework, she was to become aware of her breathing several times during work hours, and she made some interesting observations: she discovered that her breathing was very shallow most of the time, and became even more so when she looked at her co-worker, Jane, and increased her working speed to keep up with her. She also discovered that she was hardly breathing at all when her boss came into the room.

During the next session, she participated in all the exercises. Using crayons and paper was a strange experience; when she was told to draw her body, she did not know how. One of the group leaders told her just to start moving crayons on the paper, and she discovered that she had drawn a spruce tree. It looked withered, and it made her very sad to look at it. Somehow she knew that 'this is me'. When she was asked to stand on the floor and become the tree, she was aware of tension in her whole body and very shallow breathing. Again, she started crying, but she felt a little less embarrassed because she saw that some of the others, including one from her own workplace, were crying too. Listening to some of the others sharing their drawings was both embarrassing and interesting. The drawings were so different, but they all had a story to tell.

Still sceptical, Judith decided to continue in the group. She liked to write in her workbook, and she was not embarrassed any longer when listening to the others. When they shared experiences in groups of three, she even started to like telling the others about herself. Both group members and group leaders really listened to her. Now she was not only to become aware of her breathing while working, but also to be aware of muscular tension, and practice 'letting go' while she was working. Practicing to become aware of the working speed that felt right for her and her bodily reactions was very difficult, but it helped to think about the group members and know that they supported her. She had started to have lunch with the two other participants from her group some days, and they often had a good laugh when they shared situations related to doing their homework.

One of them had even dared to say 'no' when the boss had made a pass at her. With the support from her colleagues, Judith knew that she would have the courage to do the same, but she still needed more time.

When they worked with 'joy' as a theme in the group, Judith became aware that she had hardly given any time for joy in her life over the last few years, and she realized that the laughs she had with her two colleagues from the group during working hours energized her at work. Working with guilt and anger in the group was also very interesting and scary.

When she was about half way through the program, Judith started to look forward to the sessions. She cried more during some sessions than she could ever remember having done in her adult life. She discovered that she also laughed more than she had done for years. She really liked many of the group members, and now it felt good to share both her discoveries from the work in the group and experiences from the homework with the others. Their support meant much, and gave her the strength to make changes in her life, both within herself and in relation to her working and home life. She was very glad to 'still have' her two colleagues from the hospital laundry when the group ended.

Judith Smith had never written a poem before, but at the last session she read out the following:

Have I changed?
The withered spruce is gone.
Now perhaps I am a pine tree.
A bit uneven in shape and bark,
but still a sound tree.
My roots are perhaps still a bit too short.
They need a constant flow of humidity and fertilizer.
I know that I now better can endure the wears and tears of winds
    and storms.
Like a pine tree I don't change much with the seasons.
I am on my way.

Acupuncture and myofascial pain: move it all over again

Terje Alraek

Throughout the world, complementary medicine (CM) has become more and more popular. In 1997 there were more visits by Americans to CM practitioners than to primary care physicians (Eisenberg *et al.*, 1998). Acupuncture, a popular complementary therapy in the West, is used by approximately 1 000 000 Americans annually. Equal interest and increase in use of CM can be found in many other industrialized countries (Eisenberg *et al.*, 1998; Goldbeck-Wood *et al.*, 1996).

Acupuncture is a part of traditional Chinese medicine which has developed over thousands of years and has its own unique understanding, both of diseases and in prevention of diseases. Even today, traditional medicine makes up about 40% of all healthcare treatments sought in China. After President Nixon's visit to China in 1972, acupuncture was brought to the West with enthusiasm, triggered by a journalist's personal description of an operation where acupuncture was used as a form of analgesia. Due to this, a lot of research was started on acupuncture. The results showed that acupuncture had an effect on diseases where pain was a major part of the problem. This effect was mainly explained by the production of endorphins, serotonin and acetylcholine in the CNS, enhancing analgesia. Other theories as to why acupuncture can reduce pain are linked to the principles of gate control mechanisms. This seems to be the reason why we find acupuncture in a lot of pain clinics in hospitals. The explanation of its efficacy is now rooted in Western medical terms, and is therefore accepted into these hospitals, but in dealing with patients and their diseases, we still have to use the ancient theories from traditional Chinese medicine to get the full value of this therapy.

How does Chinese medicine understand myofascial pain?

In old textbooks, we find sayings like: 'Where there is pain there is an acupuncture point.' To some extent, we can say that this corresponds to the trigger-point theories, but for an acupuncturist, it is not enough to only use trigger-point acupuncture for patients with myofascial pain. Dealing with such a complicated pain syndrome, I as an acupuncturist have to use the framework given by traditional Chinese medicine to evaluate and diagnose my patients, so they can get the full advantage from this therapy. That is why I use the heading 'Move it all over again'. One concept in Chinese medicine is the movement of Qi (not equivalent to the Western concept of energy). This movement or lack of movement can take place in the acupuncture meridians, in the *zang/fu* (the naming of organ pictures in traditional Chinese medicine) or in the mind. In dealing with patients with myofascial pain, it is also of great importance to get to know where their pain is located; is it fixed or does it move around? Is the pain burning, does it feel good to be touched on the painful area or does this make it feel worse? Is the pain related to weather changes, to stress, to emotional ups and downs, and does it change according to the patient's activity? The immense tiredness some of these patients experience is also an expression of too little Qi. This can be caused by devastating pain which prohibits deep and refreshing sleep. All this information must be taken into account before the practitioner can choose the correct acupuncture points to work on. Therefore, two patients with the same Western diagnosis will receive different acupuncture treatment due to the fact that their description of how they experience their pain and how they live with it is different.

The acupuncture treatment is given once or twice a week or more, depending on the condition of the patient. After a course of 10 treatments, there should be an idea as to whether acupuncture can help or not. If there is a good response, treatments can continue in a way which the patient and the therapist are comfortable with. From my own experience as an acupuncturist, it is important not to overload these patients with good advice, whether it is evidence-based or not. A lot of these patients are given a long list of dos and don'ts by people who wish them all the best, but in the long run this can cause a lot of frustration due to not being able to follow all the advice. When acupuncture helps, the patient will slowly experience less pain and they will have more energy. Slowly, and at their own speed, they can start to listen to their own needs. Many doctors in general practice who deal with patients with myofascial pain are not sympathetic to holistic thinking and the interaction of mind and body.

Research on acupuncture

Over the last 20 years, a lot of scientific papers have been published about acupuncture and its possible effect on different diseases. From established medicine, critiques of research have mainly been that they are of low quality, and very few RCTs have been performed. Some of the research papers show little understanding or respect for traditional Chinese medicine. Too many papers include standard treatments for a disease, where one should expect a more individualistic approach to the prescription of acupuncture treatment.

Research on acupuncture and fibromyalgia

'Is acupuncture effective in the treatment of fibromyalgia?' is a recently published article with an evidence-based methodology (Berman *et al.*, 1999). The authors analyzed seven studies, only one of which was of high quality. The conclusions are, therefore, made on little material, but it is suggested that real acupuncture is more effective than sham acupuncture ('placebo') for improving symptoms in patients with fibromyalgia. More RCTs are needed to provide more robust data on effectiveness. In another small study (Sprott *et al.*, 1998), it was observed that acupuncture treatment of patients with fibromyalgia was associated with decreased pain levels and fewer tender points as measured by visual analogue scales and dolorimetry. This was accompanied by decreased serotonin concentration in platelets and an increase of serotonin and substance P levels in serum. These results suggest that acupuncture may be associated with changes in the concentration of pain-modulating substances.

The art of living with pain: recovery through acknowledgment

Kirsti Malterud

The nature of chronic disorder implies that cure may be an inadequate goal for management. However, for CMP the consequence of such an understanding is not that life is over or that increasing deterioration will happen. On the contrary, these conditions are often characterized by patterns shifting between ups and downs. The ups and downs may be more or less frequent, the amplitude between good and bad days may vary between individuals and provocative factors cannot always be predicted. Yet, there is hope on many levels that can be identified and mobilized. Although the pain disturbs the well-being and ability of the patients, their bodies are yet intact and will not be deformed, like many patients with rheumatoid arthritis or multiple sclerosis experience. Although patients with CMP may feel helpless when they are not able to maintain their everyday tasks at work or in their family, they never arrive at a state where intensive care is needed, such as with patients suffering from serious strokes or dementia.

These matters may be obvious for the physician, but are yet significant reminders in the negotiations between patient and healthcare provider, when common ground regarding the impact of the health problems is to be achieved. For this group of patients, with stories of long-term struggling to be seen and to be taken seriously by the healthcare and insurance systems, it may be hard to get excited about ups and good days. Maintaining and generating hope by stressing the strengths and resources of the individual are important contributions from the family physician, who often accompanies patients with CMP through many years. This is partially a question of attitude, and partially a question of practical action.

Recovery: coming to terms with the painful life

Chronic disorders require objectives and strategies for management which are very different from those applied in transient or curable conditions. The progress of medicine in the last couple of centuries has made people believe that any illness can be cured and that suffering is no longer necessary. In chronic pain disorders, the major challenge for both the physician and the patient is to obtain a resourceful balance between the painful realities of permanent disability and the hopeful expectations of a future life containing well-being and joy. It is about coming to terms with the consequences of illness, without being resigned to the belief that nothing can be done. The physician should be reminded that the burdens of this task are usually far more heavy for the patient, although medical school training offers limited preparation for dealing with long-term illness and witnessing the patient's continued suffering (Malterud, 2000).

In my own work with patients with CMP, I have applied some ideas about recovery that originally had been worked out by and for patients with mental illness. By presenting these, however, I would warn the reader against regarding the pain disorders as basically mental problems. The interface between CMP and mental illness is about living a life with chronic disability, rather than related etiology. In medicine, the concept of recovery has mostly been applied to medical activities in the emergency room or in the process of waking up after surgical interventions. Here, we speak about an extended understanding of recovery.

According to Anthony, the concept of recovery does not mean that the suffering has disappeared, all symptoms are removed, and/or functioning completely restored (Anthony, 1996). Recovery is described as a deeply personal, unique process of changing one's attitudes, values, feelings, goals, skills and/or roles. It is a way of living a satisfying, hopeful and contributing life even with the limitations caused by illness. Anthony remarks that successful recovery from a catastrophe does not change the fact that the experience has occurred, that the effects are still present and that one's life has changed forever. Successful recovery means that the person has changed, and that the meaning of these facts to the person, therefore, has changed.

Deegan (1996) writes about her own journey of recovery from mental illness. She underlines that the goal is not to become mainstreamed or normal, but to become the unique, awesome, never-to-be-repeated human being that we are called to be. She says that recovery does not mean cure, but rather an attitude, a stance and a way of approaching the day's challenge. Deegan describes how becoming what she calls 'hard at heart' may be a maladaptive strategy used by desperate people who are at great risk of losing hope through the burdens of chronic illness. Recovery requires an environment that opposes this strategy, where the patient is empowered to become the acting subjective, creating some new meanings of life, establishing a level of well-being in the family or at work in spite of considerable problems that are often invisible. Thesen has summarized the recovery concept as the opposite of resignation and despair; trusting the hope of a future life (Thesen and Malterud, 1998). Quoting Anthony, she lists the vital tools in the process of recovery as treatment, rehabilitation and peer support. Each of these components is supposed to support, not obstruct, the recovery process lived by the patient.

Patient-centered recovery approaches in primary care

The primary care provider cannot force recovery upon the patient. Recovery is a personal process, and a patient-centered strategy demands that the physician identifies and gives privilege to the patient's agenda so that management can enhance recovery. Seeing the patient as a whole person may help the physician realize why hope may disappear temporarily or permanently in the patient. Perhaps the structural conditions of her workplace impose pressure and loads upon her, beyond what she feels she can stand. She may not be in charge of change or control, or she may lose her health insurance by asking for alterations. Perhaps her husband repeatedly discards her, humiliates her and sometimes beats her. Her economic situation does not allow her to reflect upon divorce. The patient may be an unemployed man whose chances for a permanent job are doomed because of his pain problems, or he may feel his body betrays him and turns him into an old man, although he just turned 40. One solution may be to become hard-hearted. By eliciting the patient's agenda and understanding more of this, the physician may be aware of the need to prevent a common feeling of hopelessness, and explore and encourage the patient's strong sides and resources.

The impact of treatment, in the sense of cure, should not be overestimated. Care is often more important than cure when it comes to chronic disorders. However, talk and support can never replace the effect of specific treatment, based on a thorough physical examination, where minor components contributing to bad cycles can be identified and worked upon. Maybe one of the pains, inhabiting the patient's left shoulder, is not as unexplainable as it may initially appear, but turns out to be the symptom of a supraspinatus tendinitis. A steroid injection may provide magic relief and break a bad circle of dysfunctional pain spreading between muscle groups. An x-ray picture may portray a calcification for which surgery is appropriate. With these matters, I want to give some reminders about patient-centered care as the negotiated sum of both the patient's and doctor's agenda (Malterud, 2000). While the first one is often neglected, the second might also disappear when extensive psychosocial problems dominate. Never forget that new diseases may also appear in patients who have previously been comprehensively investigated, or that recurrent symptoms sooner or later may provide some diagnostic findings.

Rehabilitation is probably the most significant approach to pursue in primary care. Rehabilitation is much more than bringing temporarily sick or disabled people back to work; it is about rearranging the practical, physical and social life of a person who has had his or her plans or future dramatically distorted. Multidisciplinary approaches are required, with collaboration between professionals such as physiotherapists, occupational therapists, social workers, psychologists, medical specialists (most often from rheumatology or neurology) and care providers. Health insurance systems and social security officers are often involved, and sometimes the patient's employer and co-workers. To co-ordinate these efforts is usually the complex, but important task of the family physician. Overview of systems, understanding of competence within other professions, as well as communication and negotiation skills are required. In a patient-centered approach, the patient is an active participant of this collaboration network, and not an object who is being talked about by the professionals.

Peer support cannot be provided by the physician. The strength of this component is the experience of meetings among equals, sharing stories and knowledge and discussing policies and strategies for change. The family physician can contribute to this by actively encouraging the patient to join groups and organizations, and getting hold of addresses and names of contact persons. Even if the physician does not fully agree with the goals or policy of the organization, the patient should not be denied access due to disapproval or lack of information.

Judith Smith's faithful and skilled professional companion

Judith Smith trusts her family physician, although they have been struggling and fighting for years with each other about her pain. After a period of disappointing frustrations, she finally realized that he would never be able to take away her pain. He was able to tell her that this was not because he did not know what she was suffering from, and shared his confidence that no unidentified, serious underlying illness was causing the pain. She felt she was being taken seriously, and she knew he would be trustworthy regarding the sensitive matters she had confided to him about several possible sources of pain, which were still a part of her life. Last year he organized a group where a social worker and a physiotherapist visited her workplace to explore her chances of continuing working in the laundry after a period of sick leave. However, now she receives her disability pension, and joins a weekly group-based treatment program based on gentle movement and acknowledging interaction. Somehow, she feels better by recognizing that she is not the worst off in this group, and that she is able to contribute. The group is organized by the local chapter of the fibromyalgia organization. Judith knows she can always call for an appointment with her family physician, even when there is nothing new to report. Someone is there to see her, support her and accompany her through her lifelong journey with suffering and chronic illness.

References

Anthony WA (1996) Recovery from mental illness: the guiding vision of the mental health service system in the 1990s. *Psychosoc Rehab J.* **16**: 11–23.

Ashburn M and Staats P (1999) Management of chronic pain. *Lancet.* **353**: 1865–9.

Benson H, Kotch JB, Crassweller KD and Greenwood MM (1977) Historical and clinical considerations of the relaxation response. *Am Sci.* **65**: 441–5.

Berman BM, Ezzo J, Hadhazy V and Swyers JP (1999) Is acupuncture effective in the treatment of fibromyalgia? *J Fam Pract.* **48**: 213–15.

Bjordal JM and Greve G (1998) What may alter the conclusions of reviews? *Phys Ther Rev.* **3**: 121–32.

Buckelew SP, Conway R, Parker J *et al.* (1998) Biofeedback/relaxation training and exercise interventions for fibromyalgia: a prospective trial. *Arthritis Care Res.* **11**(3): 196–209.

Burton AK, Symonds TL, Zinzen E *et al.* (1997) Is ergonomic intervention alone sufficient to limit musculoskeletal problems in nurses? *Occup Med.* **47**(1): 25–32.

Chan G (1996) *Treatment of Chronic Pain: intramuscular stimulation for myofascial pain of radiculopathic origin.* Churchill Livingstone, Edinburgh.

Deegan P (1996) Recovery as a journey of the heart. *Psychiatr Rehab J.* **3**: 91–7.

Ehrmann-Feldman D, Rossignol M, Abenhaim L and Gobeille D (1996) Physician referral to physical therapy in a cohort of workers compensated for low back pain. *Phys Ther.* **76**(2): 150–6.

Eisenberg DM, Davis RB, Ettner SL *et al.* (1998) Trends in alternative medicine use in the United States, 1990–1997: results of a follow-up survey. *JAMA.* **280**: 1569–75.

Epping-Jordan JE, Wahlgren DR, Williams RA *et al.* (1998) Transition to chronic pain in men with low back pain. *Health Psychol.* **17**(5): 421–7.

Feine JS and Lund JP (1997) An assessment of the efficacy of physical therapy and physical modalities for the control of chronic musculoskeletal pain. *Pain.* **71**(1): 5–23.

Field TM (1998) Massage therapy effects. *Am Psychol.* **53**: 1270–81.

Flor H, Fydrich T and Turk DC (1992) Efficacy of multidisciplinary pain treatment centers: a meta-analytic review. *Pain.* **49**(2): 221–30.

Goldbeck-Wood S, Dorozynski A, Lie LG *et al.* (1996) Complementary medicine is booming worldwide. *BMJ.* **313**: 131–3.

Goldenberg DL (1993) Fibromyalgia: treatment programs. *J Musculoskel Pain.* **1**(3–4): 71–81.

Halpern M (1992) Prevention of low back pain: basic ergonomics in the workplace and the clinic. *Baillière's Clin Rheumatol.* **6**(3): 705–30.

Haugli L, Steen E, Lærum E, Finset A and Nygård R (2000) Agency orientation and chronic musculoskeletal pain: effects of a group-learning program based on personal construct theory. *Clin J Pain.* **16**(4): 281–9.

Haugli L, Steen E, Lærum E, Nygård R and Finset A (2001) Learning to have less pain: is it possible?: a one-year follow-up study of the effects of a personal contruct group learning programme on patients with chronic musculoskeletal pain. *Patient Educ Counsel.* **45**(2): 111–18.

Hurwitz EL, Aker PD, Adams AH, Meeker WC and Shekelle PG (1996) Manipulation and mobilization of the cervical spine: a systematic review of the literature. *Spine.* **21**(15): 1746–59.

Jacobson E (1987) Progressive relaxation. *Am J Psychol.* **100**(3–4): 522–37.

Jessup BA and Gallegos X (1994) Relaxation and biofeedback. In: PD Wall and R Melzack (eds) *Textbook of Pain.* Churchill Livingstone, Edinburgh.

Karasek R and Theorell T (1990) *Healthy Work: stress, productivity and the reconstruction of working life.* Basic Books, New York.

Kelly G (1955) *The Psychology of Personal Constructs.* Norton, New York.

Linton SJ (1994) Chronic back pain: integrating psychological and physical therapy: an overview. *Behav Med.* **20**(3): 101–4.

Malterud K (1992) Women's undefined disorders: a challenge for clinical communication. *Fam Pract.* **9**: 299–303.

Malterud K (2000) Symptoms as a source of medical knowledge: understanding medically unexplained disorders in women. *Fam Med.* **32**: 417–25.

Martin L, Nutting A, MacIntosh BR *et al.* (1996) An exercise program in the treatment of fibromyalgia. *J Rheumatol.* **23**(6): 1050–3.

Merleau-Ponty M (1996) *Phenomenology of Perception* (10e). Routledge & Kegan Paul Ltd, London, UK.

Miller W and Rollnick S (1991) *Motivational Interviewing: preparing people to change addictive behavior.* Guilford Press, New York.

NIH Technology Assessment Panel (1996) NIH technology assessment panel on integration of behavioral and relaxation approaches into treatment of chronic pain and insomnia. *JAMA.* **276**(4): 313–18.

Nordin M and Campello M (1999) Physical therapy: exercises and the modalities: when, what, and why? *Neurol Clin N Am.* **17**(1): 75–89.

Pennebaker JW (2000) Telling stories: the health benefits of narrative. *Lit Med.* **19**: 3–19.

Pennebaker JW, Hughes CF and O'Heeron RC (1987) The psychophysiology of confession: linking inhibitory and psychosomatic processes. *J Pers Soc Psychol.* **52**: 781–93.

Pennebaker JW, Mayne TJ and Francis ME (1997) Linguistic predictors of adaptive bereavement. *J Pers Soc Psychol.* **72**: 863–71.

Portenoy RK (1996) Opioid therapy for chronic non-malignant pain: a review of the critical issues. *J Pain Symptom Manage.* **11**: 203–17.

Reid W (1978) *The Task-Centered System.* Columbia University Press, New York.

Ricoeur P (1971) The model of the text: meaningful action considered as a text. *Soc Res.* **38**: 529–62.

Roy R (1992) *The Social Context of the Chronic Pain Sufferer.* University of Toronto Press, Toronto, Canada.

Sandstrom MJ and Keefe FJ (1998) Self-management of fibromyalgia: the role of formal coping skills training and physical exercise training programs. *Arthritis Care Res.* **11**(6): 432–47.

Sheon RP, Moskowitz RW and Goldberg VM (1996) *Soft Tissue Rheumatic Pain: recognition, management, and prevention* (3e). Williams & Wilkins, Baltimore, MD.

Simonsen RJ (1998) Principle-centered spine care: McKenzie principles. *Occup Med.* **13**(1): 176–83.

Sims J (1997) The evaluation of stress management strategies in general practice: an evidence-led approach. *Br J Gen Pract.* **47**(422): 577–82.

Singh NA, Clements KM and Fiatarone MA (1997) A randomized controlled trial of the effect of exercise on sleep. *Sleep.* **20**(2): 95–101.

Smyth JM, Stone AA, Hurewitz A and Kaell A (1999) Effects of writing about stressful experiences on symptom reduction in patients with asthma or rheumatoid arthritis. *JAMA.* **281**: 1304–9.

Sprott H, Franke S, Kluge H and Hein G (1998) Pain treatment of fibromyalgia by acupuncture. *Rheumatol Int.* **18**(1): 35–6.

Stensland P and Malterud K (1997) New gateways to dialogue in general practice: development of a symptom diary to expand communication. *Scand J Prim Health Care.* **15**: 175–9.

Stensland P and Malterud K (1999) Communicating symptoms through illness diaries: qualitative evaluation of a clinical method to expand communication. *Scand J Prim Health Care.* **17**: 75–80.

Stuckey SJ, Jacobs A and Goldfarb J (1986) EMG biofeedback training, relaxation training, and placebo for the relief of chronic back pain. *Perceptual and Motor Skills.* **63**(3): 1023–36.

Sunshine W, Field T, Schanberg S *et al.* (1997) Massage therapy and transcutaneous electrical stimulation effects on fibromyalgia. *J Clin Rheumatol.* **2**: 18–22.

Thesen J and Malterud K (1998) Psykiatrisk rehabilitering og kvinners helse. [Psychiatric rehabilitation and women's health: a letter from Massachusetts.] *Tidsskr Nor Laegeforen.* **118**: 936–8.

Torstensen TA, Ljunggren AE, Meen HD *et al.* (1998) Efficiency and costs of medical exercise therapy, conventional physiotherapy and self-exercise in patients with chronic low back pain: a pragmatic, randomized, single-blinded controlled trial with one-year follow-up. *Spine.* **23**(23): 2616–24.

Tsai SP, Gilstrap EL, Cowles SR, Waddel LC and Ross CE (1992) Personal and job characteristics of musculoskeletal injuries in an industrial population. *J Occup Med.* **34**: 606–12.

Turk DC and Rudy TE (1994) A cognitive-behavioral perspective on chronic pain: beyond the scalpel and syringe. In: DT Tollison, JR Satterthwaite and JW Tollison (eds) *Handbook of Pain Management.* Williams & Wilkins, Baltimore, MD.

Værøy H and Merskey H (1993) *Fibromyalgia and Myofascial Pain.* Elsevier Science Publishers, Amsterdam.

Waddell G (1998) *The Back Pain Revolution.* Churchill Livingstone, Edinburgh.

Wigers SH, Stiles TC and Vogel PA (1996) Effects of aerobic exercise versus stress management treatment in fibromyalgia: a 4–5-year prospective study. *Scand J Rheumatol.* **25**(2): 77–86.

Wyszynski MB (1997) The New York pain treatment protocol: a structured therapy approach for treating the muscular components of chronic pain syndromes. *J Back Musculoskeletal Rehab.* **8**: 109–23.

7

The challenges of chronic myofascial pain: commitment to patient perspectives

Kirsti Malterud and Steinar Hunskaar

The perception of pain is an entirely subjective experience. Acknowledging this, the pain of a person cannot be contested. Yet, interpreting the meaning of bodily pain is a common matter for discussion, negotiations and sometimes conflicts in clinical practice. In this final chapter, we summarize some of the lessons taught in previous chapters, discussing challenges raised when there is a commitment to patient perspectives.

Judith Smith's story reminds us that apparently unexplained conditions will not always remain unexplained if patients are empowered to share their knowledge with the healthcare provider.

Different levels of challenges

The physician encounters challenges on different levels. First comes the challenge of reading the medical signs, trying to identify patterns that fit into the templates of medical diagnosis, i.e. simply finding out what is wrong, or the source of the pain. In practice, this is often a question of identifying or ruling out serious conditions presenting with pain, as one out of several symptoms and findings. This may be an easy task on a home-visit to an old woman who fell four hours ago, who has pain in her left hip and an outwards rotated left leg. The condition is easily identified within the biomedical framework, no conflict appears, and the patient is admitted to hospital for surgery. Another easy task may be to find out whether a couple of days with moderate chest pain could be due to lung or heart disease.

In other cases, pain and other symptoms attributed to the musculoskeletal system are not so easily interpreted. As pointed out in Chapter 1, a confusing magnitude of names are given to such complaints, reflecting diverging opinions and a lack of consensus on what it is all about. It is also admitted that the competence in diagnosis and treatment of such conditions varies among primary care practitioners, and that skills in history-taking, clinical examination and therapeutic procedures may be improved among most of us. It is the responsibility of the patient's primary care physician to keep updated on the clinically relevant advancements in pain theory, to maintain clinical competence and to put into practice new treatment options for the good of the patient. It is our hope that this book will contribute to this.

A second challenge for the physician arises when there is no obvious disease template to match the symptoms presented by the patient. Epidemiological studies show that most doctors experience this. In such cases, the diagnostic question is not immediately or clearly answered. Interpretation of the unknown or diffusely delineated symptoms is more complicated than recognizing and remembering what you were taught in medical school. Medical practice somehow assumes that symptoms due to disease belong in orderly entities, where corresponding findings will confirm the diagnosis.

This book points out several new perspectives. Understanding of pain systems concerning CMP has grown. We know more about how long-lasting pain can develop, even without a single episode of strong, acute pain starting the process. It is interesting, and maybe surprising for some, that the experimental pain researchers in their chapter state that the sensation and experience of pain is always based on physiological processes in the nervous system, whatever we consider as 'real'. There is also increasing evidence that other symptoms often seen with CMP, like fatigue, allodynia, dysuria and sleep disturbances may be part of a multiple neuroendocrine dysfunction. Then the text looks at the biopsychosocial models of chronic pain, regarding the symptom as being related to a wide range of contextual levels. Several authors show how this way of thinking is meaningful when understanding, examining and treating chronic pain patients. Traditional 'risk factors' are discussed, but the observant reader will notice that it is no longer merely scientific speculation to assume that an illness or even a chronic organic disorder may be understood as an expression of a person's efforts to come to terms with a threatening situation or lack of personal control.

The third challenge, therefore, deals with the meeting between presumed experts; the patient, who suffers from pain and worries, and the physician who is supposed to solve the medical mystery. Realizing that the diagnostic question has no clear-cut answer, the physician must look at the additional cues provided by the patient to compile the clinical knowledge required to understand what is wrong and what can be done. Finding common ground, one of the hallmarks of the patient-centered clinical method, is vital for diagnosis as well as management. In family medicine, where patients' problems commonly differ from textbook descriptions, this is especially important but is not always an easy task, even for a physician who is committed to patient-centered care. The medical gaze may easily cut through contradictions by omitting the view of the patient. At surface level, patient perspectives sometimes appear to mess up easy conclusions, while they actually may be required to understand the complex reality of lives in pain. We hope that this book will motivate physicians and other healthcare workers to challenge some of the old myths about CMP and the patients who suffer from it, and understand more by incorporating new knowledge, perspectives and the authors' experiences into their own clinical practice.

Chronic myofascial pain: a medical matter?

Myofascial pain is a commonly occurring condition, more so in women than in men. It may be argued that such pain is just part of the burden of everyday life, and as such belongs beyond the borders of medicine. However, clinical reality and epidemiology demonstrate that a considerable proportion of patients in primary care suffer from these conditions, to an extent where their well-being and working ability are seriously affected. Most of these patients perceive their pain as bodily pain, and resist interpretations where the symptoms are given a psychological label. Conflicts commonly emerge when healthcare providers ignore patient perspectives, since no pathological signs have been observed. There often are two different conceptual worlds, one in which doctors traditionally focus on the disease aspect, and the other in which the patient sees the illness aspect of expressed ailments.

Contemporary muscle and pain physiology provide models explaining how the perception of pain is modulated or regulated, suggesting that processes in the muscle may serve as pathogenetic links between several etiological causes of pain (e.g. psychological stress or monotonous work) and the individual experience of pain. There are indications that long-standing, painful stimulation in itself may cause changes in the function of the CNS. The peripheral and central mechanisms may influence each other, and with long-lasting pain a feedback loop may develop, enhancing the pain. From a scientific point of view, CMP can no longer be exiled to the domain of psychosocial problems and labeled as 'unexplained'. However, the pain was no less real before the physiological explanations were spelled out.

The context of pain

More or less a bodily phenomenon, pain certainly belongs in the context of culture, society and identity. In some cases, painful or abusive relationships at home or at work provide obvious causal explanations, supporting an under-standing of body and mind as intimately intertwined connections in the lives of human beings. As shown in this book, feminist knowledge about gendered life conditions contributes to a more specific comprehension of the relationships between oppression and pain. Yet, explanations are complex, combining speci-fic strain and social structures as triggers for individual vulnerability. Whatever caused the patient's pain, the impact of chronic pain on everyday life, identity and relationships is considerable. Quality of care requires the physician to explore the patient's perspectives. This can only be done if the healthcare provi-der clearly acknowledges the patient's version of reality, yet maintains a second view which allows for consideration of different options.

Patient-centered medicine offers both a theoretical and practical model for being a good doctor. To meet the challenges presented by patients with CMP, one way to proceed is through structuring consultations where clues offered by patients can be explored. Failure to act on these clues may result in missing opportunities to gain insight into the illness and the full context of pain in the individual case. This book has several examples of how research findings have demonstrated the huge amount of information to be gained from the patient when the illness experience is explored, a fact well in accordance with clinical experience from individual patient–doctor relationships.

Finding common ground: approaching recovery

The action-prone physician may easily feel lost in cases where cure is not uni-formly or easily available. However, the myth that nothing can be done with CMP can be put to rest. Several modalities of medical care are available, and must be thoroughly assessed with the patient. As editors, we have presented an updated review of available treatment options, using an evidence-based approach when possible. There is still much to be done in the area of CMP. In the first place, there are very few studies available. In addition, the studies that do exist are frequently at odds with clinical experience due to their selection bias.

Several authors emphasize that the management of chronic pain patients en-tails more than offering drugs and simple procedures. Collaboration with other healthcare providers, referral to specialist care and multidisciplinary clinics may be useful in many cases. Overtreatment may also occur, however, some-times with severe consequences like drug addiction or post-operative complica-tions. On the other hand, there is a danger of being nihilistic in one's approach when encountering 'yet another' patient who seems to be trapped in a situation of no cure, chronification and pessimism.

Deciding what would benefit the patient is not a task for the physician alone. The patient-centered clinical method suggests different approaches, all of them presuming a long-lasting and continous patient–physician relationship where the patient comes to feel safe and acknowledged. Thus resignation and despair can be turned into hope and recovery. To reach this objective, maintaining an understanding of the patient as the main character of the story, is the core challenge raised by patient perspectives.

Index